THE
INGREDIENT
DIET

Valerie H. Lunden, M.A.

Disclaimer

Readers are advised to consult with their physicians or
other medical practitioner before implementing any of
the suggestions that follow.

The information contained in this book is not intended as
medical advice. The author, publishers, and/or
distributors will not assume responsibility for any adverse
consequences or liability resulting from any health or
lifestyle changes described herein.

Dedication
For my friend, Agnelo. He has
kept the faith and stayed the course,
always with a kind and caring heart.

CONTENTS

PART I

PART II

ೞಀಏ

Ingredient Diet Equation

Superior nutrition = Digestion efficiency = Weight loss + Wellness

ೞಀಏ

Part I

Healthy and Happy?

The Ingredient Diet is concerned with the role of history—not science, and specifically, how people digest food. This is both an unusual and unique historical perspective, one that questions many health concepts, and challenges how our world manages weight loss and wellness.

The ID concept has been created to help people manage illness, particularly those who are overweight, diagnosed obese, or suffer from digestive illnesses, allergies, and complexities of incurable disease.

Chapter 1

The view from above

Fat bellies and fat rear ends, bulges about the throat and face, cottage cheese thighs and wiggly upper arms—the evidence of fat accumulation is not so easy to hide. Most surprising, puckered fat pockets are found on people of all ages, even our family pets.

It is plausible that a large percentage of the population believes the way they look is not at all unusual, particularly when compared with many of the people they come in contact with, their close circle of friends, or celebrities. The question is why is it now acceptable to be a few sizes larger and several pounds heavier than it used to be?

With increasingly more body fat being accumulated it could be assumed that some aspect of our biological health is not working the way it should, or more accurately, the way it worked in the past. Has the digestion process somehow become obstructed, where it now exclusively produces body fat?

Dieting because we have to

A diet should be a straightforward way to lose weight. However, in North America, over the last seven decades, obesity numbers have continued to climb.[1] These circumstances are confusing because more people are using diets than ever before. These escalating health trends also expose a new reality, traditional diets no longer work well enough to make any statistical difference in deflecting widespread fat gain or obesity.

Perhaps the very act of dieting is no longer relevant. If it was people would know how to successfully lose weight, and more important, keep the weight off.

---

[1] See U.S. Obesity maps after Resource section.

This confusion has led to the creation of many less traditional diets, as well as a host of research and expert studies, which can be tracked as far back as the middle of the twentieth century, the same point in time when obesity numbers started to climb.

Dieting—the bigger picture

However, what would obesity numbers look like if we didn't have so many diets, would these numbers increase or decline? Observed over the past seven decades, many commercial diets have been replaced by updated versions, offering new strategies to restrict food. Most of these manipulate how much and what types of foods are eaten, but none of them focus on digestion processes—not until now.

Although the majority of these diets may have at one time proved helpful, decades later most have become obsolete, either because the dieter stopped losing weight, or because some unexpected factor prohibited the dieter from using the diet properly. In the bigger picture, whatever the diet strategy the promises of weight reduction and improved health have been less than satisfactory. These are inconsistencies affecting those who have used diets for weight loss, as well as those who have gained a substantial amount of fat weight, but never used a diet. Regardless, even with deliberate calorie, fat, and portion control, a growing percentage of the world's population remains overweight, without any consistently effective diet strategy or medical intervention available to ease this problem.

What has changed?

In combination, scientific, medical, biological, and environmental factors also appear to influence weight gain. Based on lifestyle, eating a pesticide-produced diet, or one filled with organic foods, these are all varying dietary factors. Other factors include eating too frequently, or eating more food than people ate a hundred years ago.

Perhaps the most obvious changes have been to food production. Not just how foods are made, but also how foods are regulated. Because food manufacturing standards are different from place to place and country to country, their relationship to weight and health are not always obvious. The most unmonitored of these factors is the biological quality of food, which does not compare with the biological quality of food produced a hundred years ago—or for that matter even a year ago.

Fertilizers, hormones, and additives, as well as excessive food processing, keep changing, and as a consequence, the molecular structure of food continues to change. These alterations would be obvious only to the digestion process, and when explored further, may be key to curing many modern-day health problems. These are molecular changes to the nutritional benefit of food, particularly digestive issues caused after certain altered ingredients are eaten together.

> **It appears our modern weight reduction problems are not only impacted by the amount of excess calories people consume, but also the integrity of food construction, and the inferiority of ingredient quality.**

Why digestibility matters

Because food systems are constantly evolving, how our distant forefathers digested food would be different from how people digest food today, and this is primarily because the foods eaten are biologically different. This suggests food quality and the digestion process not only impact the nutritional value of foods, but also how much nutrition will be available after digestion completes. In all cases, incomplete digestion would lead to inefficient nutrition extraction, resulting in limited nutrition distribution. This impacts all foods consumed, the types of foods selected, and the various processes the body uses to digest food.

These factors become more problematic when the digestion has to manage a wide variety of

chemically created and engineered foods, eaten at every meal, over weeks, and year after year. As a sweeping statement, the way foods are created, accompanied by overeating, results in poor digestion outcomes both during and after digestion.

Advanced systems

Modern food manufacturing systems appear to have two immediate goals: The first is to create a food surplus to feed large populations, and the second, is to increase profits by introducing enticing processed foods and unique recipe combinations. These goals have resulted in the creation of many nutrient-deficient foods, as well as foods that cause severe digestion problems, either when eaten alone, or when combined with other deficient ingredients.

Eating frequency

The final digestion-related issue, most people eat using a routine or schedule. These are events called meals, and they happen throughout the day. Meals force people to eat more food more often. In most situations this is more food then the digestion can process.

Specific to digestion complexities, the chief problem is meals made with a wide variety of complex ingredients, which require more thorough digestion. **This spotlights meals made with highly processed ingredients, (in various recipes) which after being consumed, cause batches of chemically-created additives to join together in the stomach.** Any batching of additives produces digestion slow downs, which further delays, or even stops digestion cycles from completing. An example of ingredient batching is found on page 20.

Illness evolution

Offering another sweeping statement, the influence of modern food systems bears *all* the responsibility for rising obesity and body fat overproduction. This connection not only extends to the quantity of engineered and prepared foods people eat, but also how these engineered and prepared foods become sorted, and later digested. If a single digestion cycle is interrupted, this type of biological system failure automatically triggers fat production. The outcome is uncontrollable weight gain, leading to obesity and perhaps more serious health problems later in life.

Digestion factors

If the core issue is poor digestion, which eventually leads to fat gain followed by illness, this suggests digestion must first improve before overall health can improve. This premise specifically applies to instances of incomplete digestion, where eating too many complex ingredients during a single meal, and consuming meals in close succession, produces unexpected digestion problems. **Instead of quickly completing digestion cycles and extracting valuable nutrition, the digestion becomes temporarily paralyzed after under-**

digested ingredients gather together waiting to be matched with complimentary enzymes.

Complicating matters, the expectation is enzymes will always be available to digest *all* foods during the typical digestion cycle. However, when ingredients are overly manufactured, this forces the digestion to customize enzymes. These instances produce delays and incomplete digestion, particularly if unique enzymes must be created to break down combinations of complex, chemically-created additives, pesticides, fertilizers, and hormones, which are the unreported molecular components of many modern foods.

Digestion anxiety

Under digestion happens when there are too many ingredients and not enough enzymes. This produces a system exhaustion called *digestion anxiety*. Digestion anxiety rejects ingredients the body cannot efficiently digest. When this happens frequently—as frequently as several times during a single day, the opportunities for fat making

increase.

Consequences of poor digestion

When poor enzyme-matching cycles continue for

decades, depending on the time it takes for the

metabolism to weaken, the body will eventually become

susceptible to fat gain, allergies, and illness. These would

be unpredictable illnesses and allergies, caused by

conflicted interactions between a person's unique DNA,

incomplete digestion, and the staggered digestion of

synthetic ingredients he or she has consumed over time.

There are too many illnesses to list here (see chart on page

18) but these illnesses include the most obvious, heart

disease, and perhaps not so obvious, different forms of

cancer. In addition, there is a subcategory of physical

complaints, which often go unnoticed. This list includes

common digestion counter reactions such as acid reflux,

vitamin deficiencies, colds, the flu, adult acne, and all

forms of irritable bowel syndrome.

Noticeably, the majority of these illnesses, great and small, have increased in resistance over time, many of them becoming untreatable. Specific to fat gain and obesity, these are no longer isolated concerns, but today affect overweight nations, described as global clusters of over-fat production.

Fat is the human burden

The root cause of fat buildup is the body initiating protective measures to activate a new fat bi-product. For the purposes of this program this bi-product has been named secondary fat. The build-up of secondary fat produces higher body toxicity, followed by a gradual decline in immune health.

Connected to this is the rise in numbers of obscure sicknesses—most having no definitive cures. This surge in both diseases and illnesses is curious, particularly when we live in an age where science and medicine, as well as overall cleanliness, food quality, and general living conditions, are considered advanced. As a consequence, in

12

the absence of reliable cures, obesity and many other illnesses have been labeled by science as major health threats.

Perhaps surprising, modern interventions (statistically) have not been successful in curbing or minimizing these threats. These health issues also appear more rampant in large urban hubs across the world. Coincidentally, people living in these hubs eat larger quantities of engineered foods, when compared to parts of the world where populations have less access to foods made with processed and engineered ingredients.

Chemical medicines

Diagnosing diseases and matching reliable cures will become more difficult if the digestion is constantly trying to adapt to new chemical additives. These additives are not only found in complex recipes, but also medications, either prescribed or purchased over the counter. This includes modern pain relievers, vaccines, and numerous inoculations.

13

Specific to modern medicines, depending on the severity of the disease, especially cancers, the ability to find permanent or effective cures will become less likely, particularly if the digestion and immunity both weaken at the same time. This situation becomes more serious if diseases mutate and spread, after becoming resistant to chemically created drugs.

Perhaps not anticipated, vaccines invented in the sixties and seventies are losing effectiveness, a trend that will no doubt continue as human immunity becomes further assaulted by random, synthetic, and chemically-created food additives. The faster food manufacturers use artificial means to produce new recipes, larger crop yields, and more livestock, the faster health problems will worsen.

Not just more body fat

The physical signs have already become obvious, the world's population is not only becoming progressively fatter, but also progressively sicker. For example, feeling

14

tired after eating, or getting less sleep (or too much) on a regular basis, these may be early warning signs that the body is reacting to a nutrient deficient diet. Other reactions to poor ingredient quality include bloating, burping, stomachaches, and acid reflux—all physical agitations related to poor digestion. This list also includes seemingly unrelated physical problems, including dandruff, nasal drip, and poor stool quality. To make matters worse, these conditions are often ignored, or viewed as less serious health complaints.

Biological reactions

Reducing incidences of fat gain and obesity will not be cured by simply reducing calories, controlling what categories of food people eat, or eliminating fats. These issues are related to poor digestion, or more specifically, how the body accepts and rejects molecularly altered ingredients. If the pathway to immunizing the body from fat gain and sickness requires uninterrupted and completed digestion, then paying attention to ingredient quality becomes vital to initiating permanent weight loss, as well as maintaining overall wellness.

Review: Food Manufacturing = Human Disease

During the last several decades changes to food manufacturing have advanced, allowing more chemical ingredients to find their way into ordinary foods (and medicines). These ingredients are difficult to digest, particularly when complimentary enzymes are not available to digest them.

Complicating this issue, during digestion ingredient sorting, eliminating, and storing, become further delayed. This is because synthetic additives, fertilizers, and hormones, keep changing in strength and quantity, and within a continuously changing food supply system. This happens when food manufacturers change ingredient suppliers, increase food yields, add different additives to newly-created foods, or adjust

recipe ingredients to boost profits.

ഇറ

The data presented on the following pages represents a list of illnesses, which for the most part have no permanent cures. Most surprising, these are often deadly conditions, and existing in a global environment where science and research are robust and generously funded...*It appears we have no shortage of medicines, but we do have a shortage of comprehensive cures.*

Chapter 1: Bonus video
Valerie reviews the basic concepts.
https://youtu.be/075ljUXCWRs

CAUSES OF DEATH (WORLDWIDE) - Estimates for 2000-2012				
	2000		ESCALATION 2012	
	Females Age 0-70+	Males Age 0-70+	Females Age 0-70+	Males Age 0-70+
	All ages (total) years	All ages (total) years	All ages (total) years	All ages (total) years
Nutritional deficiencies	12477	6822	14224	8405
Iron-deficiency	4932	2508	6361	3682
Malignant neoplasm	1186152	1472986	1318775	1648362
Cancer - Mouth and or pharynx	13865	47506	16733	53129
Cancer - Esophagus	15953	52898	16902	61308
Cancer - Stomach	85540	128656	72157	115396
Cancer - Colon and rectum	163194	167970	171565	192894
Cancer - Liver**	36816	68893	43849	82118
Cancer - Pancreas	68343	69636	93179	95522
Cancer - Trachea, bronchus, lung	164495	412118	214527	432780
Cancer - Melanoma and other skin	17997	22588	22730	32721
Cancer - Breast	204401	0	215641	0

Cancer - Cervix uteri	37847	0	37483	**0**
Cancer - Ovary	61920	0	**66646**	**0**
Cancer - Prostate**	0	136471	0	**157658**
Cancer - Bladder	20437	53444	**23268**	**65316**
Alzheimer's disease and other dementias	143126?	63163?	366553?	173778?
Cardiovascular diseases	3063299	2517528	2793778	2381857
Hypertensive heart disease	117644	71029	**176547**	**113257**
Stroke	1008299	652287	831094	574354
Cardiomyopathy, myocarditis, endocarditis	59567	84678	**62675**	**87560**
Respiratory diseases	248387	339335	**289366**	**360332**
Digestive diseases	212867	255059	**249854**	**297039**
Peptic ulcer disease	18310	23721	14961	20074
Cirrhosis of the liver**	62998	121410	**76974**	**137020**
Kidney diseases**	67663	63099	**92832**	**85916**
Down's syndrome	1481	1398	**1833?**	**1935?**

Illustration 1:World Health Organization (World) 2015 / See Resources for website.

*Represents the increase in disease prevalence. 100K increments.

** Represents areas of the body responsible for eliminating toxins.

[?] Represents cell distortions at the cognition level.

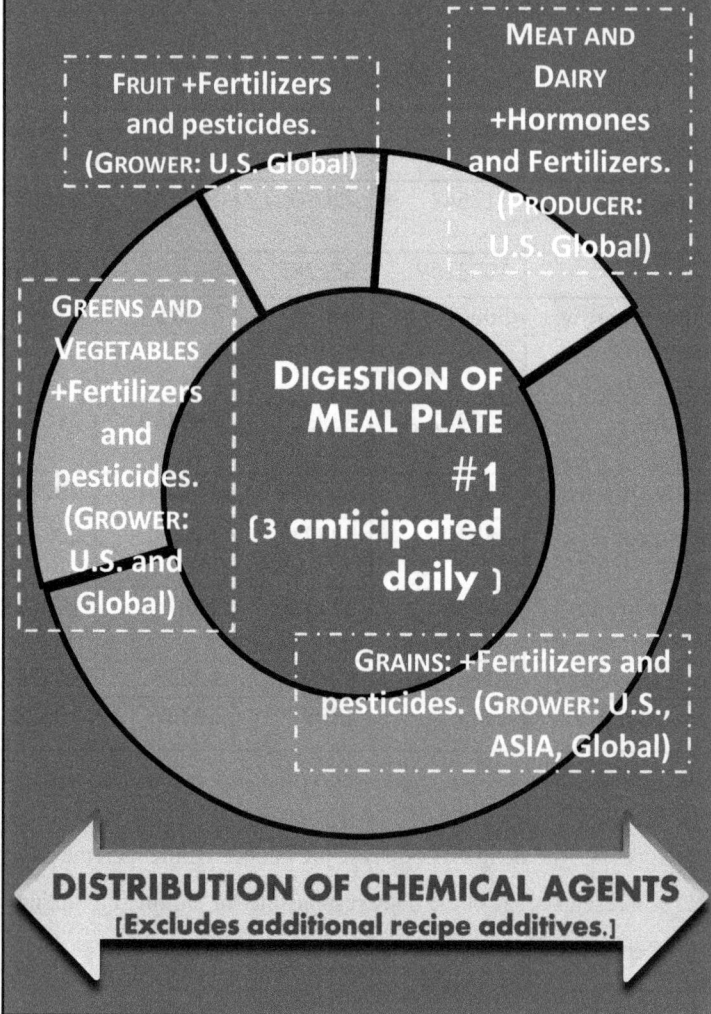

Additive distribution by plate** and country of origin

FRUIT +Fertilizers and pesticides. (GROWER: U.S. Global)

MEAT AND DAIRY +Hormones and Fertilizers. (PRODUCER: U.S. Global)

GREENS AND VEGETABLES +Fertilizers and pesticides. (GROWER: U.S. and Global)

DIGESTION OF MEAL PLATE #1 (3 anticipated daily)

GRAINS: +Fertilizers and pesticides. (GROWER: U.S., ASIA, Global)

DISTRIBUTION OF CHEMICAL AGENTS [Excludes additional recipe additives.]

*Each additive approved by various food regulatory agencies. ** One of three anticipated daily meals.

Chapter 2

Setting the Scene

> *And while smoking has been the greatest challenge of the past 20 years, it will soon be overtaken by obesity...the fastest-growing and most significant risk factor for chronic disease the nation has ever faced.*
> **America's Greatest Health Threat: Obesity**
> **Bloomberg. November, 2009**

Illness overload

An increase in worldwide digestive illnesses over time suggests the primary threat to global health could be people being diagnosed obese.[2] This is considered another negative health marker, equally as dangerous as a diagnosis of cancer, AIDS, Ebola, or Polio, where obesity

---

[2] A.M.A. Recognizes Obesity as a Disease, Ney York Times, June, 2013

could be viewed as the most dangerous disease of all humankind, particularly when the body's fat thresholds (and toxicity levels) have been crossed without a person knowing.

Why is obesity on the rise?

Obesity has become resistant to chemically engineered medicines, including cholesterol-controlling drugs, which are continually being replaced and upgraded. Gaining large deposits of body fat also appears more obvious in advanced food-making nations, where coincidentally, much of the food supply, as much as 90 percent, is in some way processed, modified, engineered, or highly refined. This includes newer food categories such as organic foods, and foods that are sold as "all natural." Ironically, even the purest of foods must be processed to maintain their "natural" state. Further curious, obesity now impacts all mean average populations, suggesting no one is immune to weight gain. This particular form of weight gain is not muscle gain, but puckered fat accumulations, substantively visible across

the entire body.

> *After being consumed, molecular changes to food, result in molecular changes within the human body.*

Problem #1: Food alterations

From the beginning of human history until

approximately 1958,[3] after food preservatives started

being regulated by the U.S. government, the biological

mechanism, and specifically the digestion, had been

exposed to very few processing changes. In contrast, the

most noticeable historical changes have been to food

integrity, taste, and texture, and the largest majority of

these alterations have happened in a relatively short

period of time, just a handful of decades.

> **Monetary cost of ingredient manipulation, U.S. 2015-16**
> *Pharmaceutical industry - 413 billion (Sales 2015)
> *Healthcare costs for obesity - $147 - $210 billion
> *Diet Industry - 64 billion dollars and rising.
> *Retail and food service sales - 5.32 trillion (Sales 2015)
> *See Reference for links.*

---

[3] *"The GRAS List" - Source: FDA.gov, see end of chapter.*

Problem #2: Eating behaviors

In centuries past the desire to eat food was instinctive, and people ate only when they were hungry. Eating routines have evolved, installing prescheduled events revolving around the timing of breakfast, lunch, and dinner. These routines are mostly behavioral, and are further influenced by lifestyle, business schedules, prescription drug instructions, and unstoppable food marketing.

Robotic food rituals, eating without appetite, and consuming too many overly processed ingredients, have altered food sensitivities. The major culprit is the large quantities of engineered foods a person eats, which over time could result in taste distortions, otherwise known as cravings. By following socialized eating behaviors, and becoming susceptible to cravings, a person will eat more food, and eat when there is no physical requirement for either energy or nutrition.

Problem #3: The 2 major fat disorders

Unlike most diets, which focus on calorie restrictions or unusual eating practices, The Ingredient Diet is concerned with reducing a condition called **Digestion Anxiety** or DA. In recent times DA could be viewed as the underlying cause of obesity, typically manifesting as large accumulations of fat across the length and breadth of the body.

Decreasing DA requires understanding the role of food manufacturing. This also requires exploring the historical complexities of food distribution from production to digestion—and equally relevant, the impact of those digestion disorders, which accelerate digestion anxiety. By examining how ingredients interact after they are consumed, may offer clues as to why overly processed foods cause digestion issues, and in some situations, indirectly contribute to a large number of incurable illnesses.

Stopping the frequency of digestion anxiety would

require interrupting new fat production—not just body fat, but also a new phantom fat substance called **Secondary Fat**. This new fat is more dangerous than natural body fat because it is difficult to digest, and accumulates in the deepest recesses of the body, making it difficult to access and remove.

ဆ ଓଷ

Improving fat loss

The Ingredient Diet is not focused on reducing the numbers on a scale. However, if there is sufficient fat loss, weight loss would be a natural outcome. Instead, The Ingredient Diet introduces a dietary system focused on reducing dangerous accumulations of body fat, both new and old. This process also requires understanding why secondary fat is different from natural body fat, knowing where and why it accumulates, and perhaps most significant, how illnesses become unavoidable when this fat accumulates in batches in remote regions of the body.

Fat overload

If fat can deposit across the entire body, this suggests that at some point during our human biological evolution something changed, something so significant it forced the digestion to produce and store more fat. For those afflicted with weight gain, this is fat-making revved up into high gear, where toxic fat, versus energy fat, is produced so quickly, and in such large quantities, it must be stored in other than the customary places.

These are biological processing inconsistencies, which require taking a closer look not only at how modern foods contribute to body fat overproduction, but also to speculate which processes the digestion uses to break down molecularly-altered foods.

Come and get it!

Although the digestion mechanism has not changed in centuries, robotic food behaviors have become common. Perhaps the most significant change to food management is not just what people eat, but how

27

frequently they eat. This spotlights a point in time when eating became associated with a timed routine, specifically, eating three meals a day.

Eating routines were started by affluent societies during the Victorian era. This novelty allowed people to eat at predetermined intervals of time, and all day long, overriding natural hunger. Unfortunately, this mostly stylistic approach to eating, called **clock eating**, involves consuming large batches of food, irrespective of whether the digestion is ready to accept a new meal cycle.

Meal evolution and genetics

Clock eating became more popular after World War II, when a decline in global economies produced a severe food shortage. Rationing, or isolating foods by meal type, helped stretch a sparse food supply, which was needed to feed large and clustered populations living in war-plagued countries.

Meal structure and composition have evolved over the decades, and as a result of clock eating, could be

28

the cause of many modern-day health problems, both noticeable and chronic. Also significant, portion sizes and plate sizes have increased, and this may be connected to post war lack progressing into modern day prosperity. Unfortunately, when there is more food consumed, this extra food would also require sorting, enzyme management, and nutrition distribution. The major concern is continuous and longer digestion cycles, particularly when chemically-created ingredients are consumed frequently, become under-digested, and as a consequence, linger in the digestion tract waiting to be expelled as waste. Remaining in the body, these poorly digested ingredients accumulate in batches, delaying the digestion times of all sequential meals.

Genetic GMOs

The frequency of clock eating, and any corresponding digestion inefficiencies, may pose threats to human genetics. In this hypothetical example incomplete digestion and bouts of digestion anxiety, would be followed by reduced nutrient distribution, happening across decades. As a gradual progression, this could cause various forms of DNA augmentation. These mechanical interruptions expose a new threat—*generational biological failure*, where without enough nutrients, the body's immunity weakens over time and becomes susceptible to genetic abnormalities. These circumstances worsen if the recipes consumed are made with different combinations of biologically unfit ingredients.

ID Program Concept

1. Almost everything consumed via the mouth must undergo a digestion cycle before nutrients and medicines can be distributed to other body systems.

2. When fewer ingredients are matched with complimentary enzymes, fewer nutrients will be extracted.

Recipes

Digestion becomes less efficient when groupings of overly processed ingredients gather together in the digestion system. These are food components made with chemically created additives, hormones, and preservatives, which must be matched with complimentary enzymes before they can move to the next phase of digestion. If clock eating happens as frequently as every four to six hours, the digestion will slowdown every time enzyme-matching cycles are interrupted. These conditions become further aggravated when customized enzymes are needed to break down stronger hormones and additives. In this scenario, any unmatched ingredients would always remain under-digested, particularly when customized enzymes cannot be created during the typical digestion cycle. The frequency of shortened digestion cycles leads to fewer nutrients being extracted, and the vast majority of under-digested ingredients being converted to secondary fat and stored.

Food evolution

Because the foods people eat today are structurally different from the foods eaten a hundred years ago, or for that matter even a month ago, how modern food systems are designed could be considered one of the greatest threats to human evolution. From state to state and country to country, dairy, vegetables, meat, grains, and fruit, are now produced using a wide variety of different standards. These differences have allowed for the creation of larger food yields, molecularly-altered foods, and unmonitored ingredient combinations, all reaching consumers in record time. **These trends may be connected to poor government oversight; specifically, a general lack of understanding of the spectrum of biological impacts, which happen every time synthetic and engineered ingredients are forced to digest together.**

More problematic, whenever processed foods are exported across state lines or to other countries, their shelf life must be artificially extended, and this requires stronger chemicals, fertilizers, and preserving agents. These complexities make it next to impossible to monitor ingredient interactions, and as a consequence, overall biological integrity.

Chemical tastes

The first indicator of poor health is reduced taste objectivity described as cravings. Being drawn to cravings is dangerous to the digestion because the foods that create these cravings are usually made with molecularly altered ingredients.

Cravings become more acute when manufacturers group certain ingredients together to create new recipes, manipulate flavors, or extend a recipe's shelf life. When eaten frequently, or in combinations, these recipes produce negative digestion interactions. These interactions are usually unpredictable, and at some point cause different physical manifestations, including allergies, infrequent bowel movements, poor stool quality, asthma, leaky gut issues, balding, irritable bowel syndrome, ulcers, sleep apnea, early menopause, low sex drive, and infertility. This is a short list of modern health concerns, which were not so prevalent fifty years ago. Many of these afflictions affect people of all ages starting from infancy with babies experiencing severe gas, to older children being diagnosed with Attention Deficit Hyperactivity Disorder. These physical reactions increase in severity as a belabored digestion causes the immunity to weaken, initiating new and unexpected health issues. Because the digestion is indirectly responsible for supporting the entire body, these problems will vary, and may include mind degenerative diseases, bone loss, joint pain, lower back pain, neurological diseases, and heart-related conditions.

Digestion under attack

Being one of nature's finest creations, the digestion tries to fend off toxin invasion by rejecting poor-quality ingredients. However, faced with having to digest too many ingredients at once, as well as managing continuous meal cycles, the digestion is unable to meet these objectives. Much worse, these interruptions result in fewer nutrients being extracted and distributed, causing the body's immunity to weaken.

To limit the impact of undigested toxins, the body's immediate reaction is to prematurely halt digestion cycles and transport all under-digested food towards the liver. This food is converted to the fat-like substance secondary fat. Secondary fat is a theoretical descriptor for a biological intervention. This is a unique storage device created specifically to house under-digested toxins. Because this topic is linked to digestion efficiency, the influence of secondary fat will be described in more detail during the next several chapters.

The progression of human weight gain

Prior to the Victorian era eating freshly prepared food was more common than it is today. Processed foods debuted during a period of time when there was rapid urbanization—an urbanization that clustered people worldwide for economic benefit. In the United States this style of urbanization is more active after long periods of war end, resulting in a sequence of aggressive industrial and social transitions. These transitions often begin with industrialization, followed by the creation of temporary housing, which allow towns and cities to quickly emerge. This also triggers population migration, deliberately moving people towards these newer towns and cities.

Specific to these deliberate migratory patterns, over time the processed food fervor has been encouraged by the vast topography and rural landscape of the United States. This vastness has clustered large groups of people in remote areas, and made it necessary to transport sustainable food across longer and longer distances.

The earliest of these large-scale migratory patterns started after the American Civil War, a time known as Reconstruction (1865–1877). This was a period of explosive infrastructure and migratory expansion, requiring more food to be transported across vast distances, from farms to newly organized towns. This could be viewed as the historic starting point of long distance food exportation in North America.

36

Dietary urbanization is just one of several simultaneous historical events encouraging rapid food evolution. Another event, and perhaps the most influential, was the building of the Union Pacific and Central Pacific railway systems. The completion of these railways in 1869, allowed for faster population migration across the country.

The railway also allowed merchandise transportation across state lines, shipping materials, clothing, and batched foods, to the towns and larger communities housing the railway workers and their families. These were often remote and clustered communities, which grew sporadically, creating an immediate demand for large quantities of nonperishable food. These foods not only had to arrive at their given destination with minimal spoilage, but also not quickly perish.

Food conservation

Pies, pancakes, and biscuits, used up leftover meat

and dairy products, which otherwise would have spoiled. Beyond using salt for pickling vegetables and smoking meats, these new foods offered the most widespread approach to localized food preservation. As more unique ingredients became available, newer recipes were invented. These locally inspired creations were also adapted whenever certain ingredients became scarce or unavailable, and this produced recipe variations from region to region.

Inventing newer recipes also encouraged food promotion in the railroad towns, where workers had more discretionary income to spend, and purchasing novelty foods became something to eagerly anticipate. This trend has continued over time, but today is far more influential, allowing for the aggressive promotion of higher resistance recipes, particularly fast foods, which reach billions of consumers worldwide.

What is tasty?

Over the centuries these ingredient manipulations

have altered our taste preferences and produced cravings for nutritionally deficient foods. These influences could be described as the customization of taste sensitivities, and would be unique to each individual because of genetic differences. Historically, these customizations have also allowed for changes to food flavor and texture, and as a consequence, increased food demand.

In pioneer times, as new clustered communities grew, and people became more settled (the Settlers) this allowed for more ingredient-rich foods to reach new and remote townships. Today there are thousands of popular (and altered) recipes in circulation, including yogurts, cereals, ice creams, potato chips, sodas, and other overly processed foods. Because these foods have artificially extended shelf lives, they are more accurately classified as hybrid varieties of fast food.

In recent decades these migratory patterns have spread across foreign borders, allowing higher resistance, multiple-ingredient foods, to become available in distant countries. As a consequence, large and clustered communities have become exposed to recipes with lower levels of digestible nutrition, more overly refined foods, and hundreds of ingredients created with different and combined chemicals. Ironically, if these engineered foods became less available, millions of people would suffer starvation. These are circumstances where large and clustered populations would have limited access to farms or other reliable sources of food. Similar food shortages have occurred throughout history, but would have greater impact today because of the sheer size, density, and remoteness of urban clusters. These constraints would limit access to the most nutritious foods first, causing them to become immediately scarce.

A thousand words

From pictorial history (mainly obtained from museum art) people in western societies began gaining fat weight in the late fifteenth century. However, more aggressive fat accumulation began after World War II

40

(post 1945).

After the war a global food shortage impacted countries with severely weakened economies and devastated farmlands. With no reliable food delivery system, something had to be done to feed millions of people, particularly those displaced by the war and forced to live in large towns and cities. These food shortages not only affected Europe, but also the United States, where servicemen were returning home to a less vibrant economy.

Grains and dairy, the modern staples, were the first ingredients to become scarce. This fueled the need to quickly produce larger quantities of faster growing and higher resistance foods. These circumstances also supported the widespread use of chemicals in fertilizers and preserving agents, which in modern times has led to the engineering of many new foods and recipes. These chemical enhancements represent the starting point of the most aggressive form of food manipulation ever seen in

41

human times.

Food preservation

Today the combining of engineered ingredients in recipes is often deliberate, and implemented not only to stimulate taste sensations, but to artificially extend the shelf life of many foods, which otherwise might quickly perish. These are specially designed foods, intended for distribution to highly populated areas, where fresh foods are often viewed as inconvenient when compared to processed foods. Coincidentally, these are also parts of the world where food selections are guided by taste preferences and the timing of meals.

Chemical preservation evolves

The earliest known preservative is salt, which has always been relatively cheap, accessible, and available in large quantities. Salt has been used to smoke and pickle food, two of the earliest preserving techniques. Today smoking and pickling, as well as other preserving techniques use chemical additives. These additives can preserve food for longer durations, not limited to weeks, but months and years.

Most of these preserving methods allow manufacturers to resell their products to secondary retail markets, particularly when they don't sell as well as expected during the first phase of distribution. In certain situations the batching of additives and preservatives allows sell by dates to be extended. In various segments of the food industry this has become a common practice, particularly if foods have to be transported across distant borders, both domestic and international. The longer a sell by date, the more likely a recipe will include heat treated fats, hormone-created meats, salt, chemical preservatives, different sugars, and bulking agents.

Illness faster!

Certain overly processed recipes, chock-full of engineered ingredients, have become famous. These fast foods did not exist a hundred years ago, but today are socially accepted. In general, fast foods are promoted as improvements, helping people save time and money. However, as governments worldwide engage in more global trading, further exposure to overly preserved foods could further threaten human health, and more so for those living in urban clusters, where these nutritionally vacant fast foods are found in abundant supply.

Digestion on/off switch

Statistically, as little as 5 percent of people who lose weight crash dieting will maintain the weight lost. This is a poor success ratio for the United States, which has a growing 64 billion dollar weight loss industry. These statistics would no doubt be higher after factoring in the negative impact of poorly digested foods.

The human digestion, being one of the most intelligent organic systems on our planet, was not designed to break down the many engineered oils, sugars, and too numerous to list, hormones, pesticides, and fertilizers. **During a single meal, literally hundreds of**
44

modified ingredients join together, waiting to be

digested. The digestion is responsible for identifying,

sorting, and ultimately breaking down all of these

elements. This process becomes further complicated

when there are multiple and continuous cycles of

breakfast, lunch, dinner, and snacks.

Poor digestion consequences

When recipes with augmented ingredients are

consumed regularly, the first and most serious biological

concern is digestion-processing confusion, closely

followed by digestion anxiety. The stronger the preserving

ingredients (usually chemically created) the more likely the

digestion will become unstable, and unable to manage,

monitor, and distribute, those nutrients needed to bolster

the immunity. This could be compared to a form of

chemical exposure, perhaps as lethal as dropping a nuclear

bomb over a large urban area. **However, this type of**

exposure is more sinister, because these chemicals

meet and clash within the body, and the adverse

health consequences would not be immediately obvious.

Digestion confusion happens when the correct enzymes cannot be matched with chemically created additives. If the digestion is unable to find or create enzymes, this results in partial digestion, followed by unmonitored toxic buildup. This leads to the activation of secondary fat production. If these digestion slowdowns happen multiple times during a single day, and continue for weeks and decades, toxic fat collects, waiting for digestion to resume at some future point—which may never happen.

Based on these concepts, eating chemically derived ingredients is physically injurious. The initial biological response may be subtle, and might even go unnoticed. The most obvious physical reactions include cravings, uncontrolled fat gain, allergies, bloating, acid reflux, water retention, stomach pains, and with much more frequency, burping, gas, and irregular stool elimination. These are early warning signs of digestion anxiety, leading to chronic illness exposure, which could happen at any time.

Review: History tells us why

A combination of taste, manufacturing, and geographical influences have supported the growth of a sprawling food supply system needed to feed remote and clustered populations. This has also allowed the processed food industry to gain considerable momentum over the decades, and food ingenuity to become vital to not only avoiding food spoilage, but feeding isolated groups of people.

Based on historical trends, accelerated fat gain could be viewed as a severe biological counterattack, caused by ingesting different chemically engineered ingredients in batches, and over long periods of time. **This involves hundreds of different foods altered at the molecular level, which decades later produces different reactions at the cellular level in the human**

body. This could also be the starting point of the body's inability to properly digest food, potentially leading to the most dangerous of all health-related issues, the harvesting of secondary fat—a protective mechanism used by the organic body to isolate the adverse effects of toxic buildup.

These poor digestion outcomes have become more debilitating over time, particularly when newer innovations in seed germination and the genetic modification of livestock now play a prominent role in food manufacturing. These chemical augmentations have infiltrated almost all food systems worldwide, and spanning four generations, may be responsible for producing chronic sickness, as well as adversely altering human genetics. Because of these varying food production issues, an influential processed food industry, with little global regulation, has contributed to our current health crisis.

The combining of engineered and overly

48

processed foods (and chemically-derived medications) cause harm to the human digestion, producing the most dangerous of all physical reactions, the digestion's inability to extract nutrition from the foods eaten. This problem is further aggravated when groupings of engineered ingredients cluster together in periodic succession during clock eating, and inside the most active and perpetuating system of the body—the digestion.

℘℃ Q

Chapter 2: Bonus video
Valerie discusses Secondary Fat.
https://youtu.be/56z73WvjGSw

Certain historic food legislation could be linked to the deterioration of worldwide food quality. This particular legislation (below) could be the starting point of modern-day digestion problems.

1958 Food Additives Amendment

Congress recognized that many food substances would not require a formal premarket review by FDA to assure their safety, either because:

- o Their safety had been established by a long history of use in food; or
- o By virtue of the nature of the substances, their conditions of use, and the information generally available to scientists.

- Two-step definition of "food additive:"

- o Broadly includes any substance that becomes a component of food or otherwise affects the characteristics of food.

- o Excludes substances that are recognized, among qualified experts, as having been adequately shown through scientific procedures (or, in the case of a substance used in food prior to January 1, 1958, through experience based on common use in food) to be safe under the conditions of their intended use.

December 9, 1958: FDA published a list of GRAS substances and incorporated the list in Title 21 of the Code of Federal Regulations.

"The GRAS List" - Source: FDA.gov

Chapter 3

Fat or obese, who decides?

> Our modern health problems are not just related to the excess calories and fat people consume, but in combination, to the inferiority of modern food construction—and as an unforeseen consequence, inadequate nutrition distribution over time.

In 2013 the American Medical Association classified obesity as a disease. This direction is significant because this could result in future legislation allowing physicians to more readily prescribe drugs to correct obesity. Such legislation could also offer insurance companies an avenue to scrutinize obesity-related medical claims, and as a consequence increase premiums. Last but not least, pharmaceutical companies would profit by introducing newer, but grossly inadequate chemically derived medications and vaccines, which is already happening. These drugs would have higher potencies, and as a result cause more harm than good to the digestion.

Finally, certain obesity classifications may already influence how those suffering from increased weight gain are medically identified, how medical information and data are collected, and how using this data could segregate those who have become obese after suffering from severe nutrient deficiencies.

Dieting—so far, it doesn't work

Modern weight-loss solutions, which encourage eating diet foods, taking diet pills, or undergoing surgical procedures to block the digestion, may have helped a few people become less obese, however, none of these strategies have solved or even reduced worldwide obesity statistics.

Overall, the direction of dietary science has been stagnant. A revolving door focused on reinventing weight reduction products, adapting shakes and supplements,

upgrading diabetes and cholesterol-controlling drugs, and

introducing a host of haphazard research projects—none

offering permanent solutions. Most important, and

specific to obesity, the unanswered question remains, why

does body fat easily accumulate across the *entire* body?

A rebellion against convention

The Ingredient Diet begins a fat rebellion. This

rebellion reevaluates uncertain scientific theories and

misguided pharmacology, which, in the opinion of this

body of work, appear out of touch with our present-day

fat-making crisis. Interesting to note, *pharmacology* comes

from the classic Greek *Pharmakon*, meaning "poison," and

Logia, the "knowledge of."Today the knowledge and use

of chemicals in foods and medications is overly popular,

as well as complex. However, what remains consistent is

the instructions for a wide range of prescription drugs,

which require consuming food, and utilizing the digestion

and enzyme systems to absorb large combinations of

chemicals into the bloodstream. However, what happens when customized enzymes are not on hand to complete digestion, or the chemically-created foods these drugs interact with produce new digestion complications? This leads to yet another unanswered question, do obesity-specific and other drugs increase toxin buildup in the body—enough to further block nutrient absorption?

Finding absolute cures

During the last three decades absolute cures have not been discovered for many serious global health issues. For example, obesity statistics have not been eased,[4] even with access to diets, drugs, surgeries, and regular exercise. Also, none of these efforts have helped the greater population manage weight gain, particularly those living in large urban clusters.

Specific to these efforts, many newly-created cholesterol controlling medications have not proved

---

[4] See U.S obesity maps after Resource section

reliable, particularly when used as long-term treatments. Some of these drugs are often stronger variations of similar products, or administered in higher doses to maintain results. Offering another insight, this paradox may be connected to seeking government approvals, where drug makers follow biologically inaccurate guidelines, and invent unstable and poorly interacting drugs. Although the speed of drug development may allow manufacturers to increase profits, this also ensures inadequately tested products reach consumers in record time.

Instead of curing symptoms of ill health, the vast majority of these drugs accelerate the placement and frequency of chemical ingredients entering the digestion. This leads to the most obvious question, why are drugs continually changing, but not curing? The answer may have some connection to why modern diets have not been consistently reliable.

Global sickness

In recent times newer health problems have surfaced, including longer durations of colds and the flu. In certain situations the flu virus has evolved to where it is now considered a life-threatening illness. Severe flu epidemics have forced governments to offer free vaccinations to reduce both the number of annual fatalities and mitigate the financial burden of illness. However, as human death tolls rise, even the most potent of vaccines is no longer reliable.

But as with diets, what would happen if we did not have vaccines? In fact, what would our global health spectrum look like if the world's medical advancement were not the best they have ever been?

> **Ironically, more and different chemicals are needed to heal the adverse effects of those chemicals already being used to create the global food supply.**

In less advanced nations, where overly processed foods are eaten less frequently, the flu and common cold, as well as incidences of obesity and cancer, are less common threats[5]. Coincidentally, these are also countries where chemically created medications are less available. This may be because illnesses are more likely to occur from environmental impacts, poverty, and a lack of basic needs.

Dieting differences

The authors of certain modern diets have introduced unique and unconventional approaches to tackling excess weight gain. One of these methods is high-protein diets. These programs attempt to replicate what our prehistoric ancestors ate by introducing different ways to increase dietary protein. Unfortunately, this premise fails to consider how the continuous reengineering of our

---

[5] Almost 50% of people hospitalized for the flu are obese| Weise, USATODAY, January 13, 2014

present day food supply, as well as any possible reduction in nutritional value that results, bears no comparison to the protein sources eaten in prehistoric times. Based on these changing factors, promoting a high-protein diet because it is similar to what our (very) distant ancestors ate is simply unrealistic.

Our prehistoric ancestors also had different and fewer food choices than we have today. Mass-manufactured foods such as chicken, pork, lamb, beef, dairy, and wheat, were not available. Instead, they ate foods not remotely comparable such as game (buffalo, venison, bison) and vegetation versus vegetables. Specific to food under refinement, many of those original ingredients may have had a higher digestion integrity, and as a consequence, a higher nutritional value.

One surprising constant is the alignment of the human teeth, which has changed very little. This suggests our ancestors were most likely meat eaters, although flesh foods would have been a luxury item, and eaten less

58

frequently. A nomadic lifestyle prohibited consuming meat every day, and certainly never three times a day. Regular hunting was also not possible because of changing climates and terrains. If there was fresh meat to eat, it was usually eaten immediately, and almost always undercooked. Food access was also restricted by geography, climate, season, and most relevant, scarcity. All of these issues offer a more realistic explanation as to why our ancestors ate less food, and probably less protein then we do today.

Environmental constraints also distinguished our distant (prehistoric) ancestors as people who roamed the land, versus settling in one place. This forced them to forage for whatever food they could find. Leading a nomadic lifestyle meant fresh meat could not be stored, transported, or preserved. The biological benefits of eating freshly killed and undercooked meat would have offered an enzyme-compatible source of food, been digestion friendly, and quickly met both nutrition and energy requirements.

These circumstances also suggest the largest amount of food was probably eaten once a day. This would have allowed time for the digestion to complete all of its various processes, thereby reducing incidents of indigestion, fat making, and waste accumulation. This could be why toxins, whatever few there were, easily passed out of the body, and were never stored. As mentioned, our ancestors faced many environmental dangers, and may have even succumbed to food poisoning on occasion, but in general, digestion was a smoother, less obstructed process. As their lifestyle permitted, they ate less food, and more fresh food. Eating events were also less frequent—and there was certainly no clock eating.

Perhaps stating the obvious, there was also no processed or preservative-rich foods in their diet. All of these factors suggest there was less food to eat, less food

60

to digest, and the majority of foods eaten were highly enzymatic, meeting all biological and digestive requirements. With limited food variety, our ancestors were forced to adapt to a vegetarian lifestyle—this was certainly not by choice. This also allowed for eating more vegetation versus vegetables, because agrarian and garden farming had not yet been invented.

Their diet would also have been devoid of grains and dairy. These foods could only be created if people settled on the land or managed animals. Instead, grains and dairy would have been inconvenient foods because they were too difficult to create, too difficult to store, and too cumbersome to prepare. Finally, nuts and fruit (mostly berries) would have been eaten fresh off the bush. These were seasonal foods, available only in certain areas, and at certain times of the year.

Our ancestors lived in conditions of extreme food purity and scarcity, a circumstance incomparable with our gargantuan food manufacturing systems and unprecedented food abundance. Scarcity provided less food, but these foods had a higher nutritional and digestive value. Their taste buds were also less refined, making the consuming of foods mostly instinctive; they were also not entranced by cravings. The ease of digestion allowed for accelerated nutrient absorption, possibly helping our ancestors stay healthier and live longer. These advantages do not exist today, particularly when food manufacturing is deliberate, and recipes are designed to induce cravings, ensure repeat purchases, and boost manufacturer profits.

Overall, our ancestors lived an unpredictable lifestyle, where food consumption, combined with overall digestion performance were influenced by many factors, including changing environments, difficult weather patterns, food scarcity, and most important, non-existent food engineering.

Modern digestion

Not transparent is the relationship between modern diets, altered foods, and the evolution of the digestion. Because this book offers a historical, rather than a science-based perspective on dieting, this topic will be discussed briefly.

As more combined and adulterated ingredients are consumed, it could be argued that the very act of digestion has been forced to evolve, and this has allowed the breakdown of a wider variety of chemicals, hormones, and preservatives. This has also produced an unexpected outcome—poor digestion, followed by reduced nutrition distribution, which may offer one explanation as to why in certain situations, and over time, the human digestion would be less likely to efficiently co-manage physical health. This is more accurately described as digestion failure, where the burden of matching enzymes with chemical additives produces sorting and processing delays. These inefficiencies may be why more people are being diagnosed with random and different health issues, including incurable diseases.

Diet failure

Another stylistic issue, modern diets are often designed to accommodate clock eating. Some of these programs go so far as to promote prepackaged foods and processed frozen meals—all made with engineered ingredients and chemical additives. Although these diets may initially produce weight loss, a gradual reduction in digestible nutrition triggers unexpected cravings, causing diets to fail and become less popular over time.

Dieters have also embraced diets offering enticing comfort foods made with highly refined and processed ingredients. These diets are often promoted as being delicious, time-saving, and capable of easily maneuvering social and work schedules. However, when these programs fail, dieters often blame themselves, not aware that this is not all their fault, and digestion factors are at play. These factors include the cravings produced after

64

eating large quantities of engineered and refined ingredients, and after doing so, leaving the body with an unreliable source of overall nutrition. Making matters worse, these cravings may continue long after the diet ends, suggesting weight gain would be inevitable.

> **Although cravings are usually linked to emotional reactions, what if carvings are triggered when the body does not receive enough digestible nutrition?**

Nutrition deficiencies

Not just obesity, but other modern illnesses have garnered attention after an increase in reported fatalities. Heart disease, high cholesterol, elevated blood pressure, sleep apnea, stomach ulcers, and irritable bowel syndrome, are a short accounting of many severe and undertreated health issues. The list on the next page includes more serious illnesses, which similar to the previous examples have no permanent cures. Based on the theories expressed in this body of work, these illnesses may be connected to decades of inadequate nutrient absorption, eventually causing the body's immunity, genetics, and sensory systems, to decline.

Cancer	ALS
Dementia	Shingles
Fibromyalgia	Alzheimer
Obesity	Arthritis
Diabetes	Melanomas
Asthma	Endometrioses
Parkinson's	Tumors (all types)

Documented illnesses with no permanent cures.

Cut and tuck approach

Beyond dieting, the newest weight loss innovations include surgical procedures. These surgeries block the digestion, subsequently forcing the appetite into submission. For the obese dieter these efforts may be a last resort, ventured into after a string of many failed diets. Because these procedures are expensive, they have not been accessible to the vast majority of people who are overweight. Regardless, any overall health benefits (after surgery) would be undermined if lifelong eating behaviors did not change, and digestible nutrition continued to be absent from the overall diet.

Dieting ironies

Individuals who diet regularly may have become yo-yo dieters. Cycles of losing and gaining weight have caused cravings to become triggered and diets to be abandoned. As an unforeseen consequence, any weight lost is regained after the diet ends. This may have more to do with changes to food quality over time, where a gradual reduction in digestible nutrition alters taste sensitivities, advances cravings, and causes people to eat more food.

If by chance a diet yields favorable results, in the vast majority of cases any weight lost would be temporary or not maintainable, particularly after conventional eating behaviors resume. Instead, dieters might have more success if they eliminated overly processed recipes and foods, particularly foods made with nutritionally vacant ingredients.

As cravings intensify

Regularly consuming augmented and overly processed foods may create a dissatisfaction for nutritious foods, which are often avoided or abandoned when cravings intensify. The typical sequence of events begins with the diet failing, the weight lost being regained, followed by extra body fat being accumulated over time. This in turn creates a digestion environment where toxin levels become dangerously elevated, followed by the unfortunate development of unexplainable illnesses, which depending on the overall health of the immunity, could happen at any time.

There is no remedy or prescription, which can replace digestible food and high-quality nutrition. **Because the digestion is a self-healing organic system, if caught in time, there may be an opportunity to reverse negative health conditions,**

68

allowing many, if not all adverse health issues to improve. But this can only happen when enough high quality nutrients are added back into the diet, and in large enough quantities where the body can repair and heal itself.

ଛୀଓଙ

Startling facts

These are food-related issues that often go unnoticed.

- Many people in the United States have access to FDA-approved foods and drugs, however, the United States remains the fattest and sickest country in the world (per capita).

- People in the United States have access to affordable and high-quality organic fruits and vegetables, however, the United States remains the fattest country in the world (per capita).

- More people in the United States than anywhere else worldwide, participate in exercise programs a minimum of three times a week, however, the United States remains the fattest country in the world (per capita).

- Even with many dietary tools and resources available, including medical and scientific intelligence, permanent cures do not exist to eradicate obesity, cancer, or premature dementia. Furthermore, vaccinated diseases such as chicken pox and polio, viewed as once cured, have resurfaced, and are making an aggressive comeback.

- Incidents of the flu and the common cold were once considered ordinary health events, however, there have been more frequent outbreaks of these sicknesses in advanced western hemisphere nations. These are disease strains, which have grown stronger and more lethal during the last several decades.

₧₨

Chapter 4

Eating toxins voluntarily

> The issue is not just ingredient inferiority, but what happens after ingredients join together in the body, are digested, and create toxic fat.

Digestion of the past

Prior to modern recipe innovations people ate more single-ingredient meals. Eating also involved fewer than five ingredients, for example, bread and butter, or grilled meat and millet porridge. These combinations had simple structures and were devoid of hormones, pesticides, and chemical additives. The ingredients that made these foods were also quickly identified and metabolized by the digestion. These foods were often bland, and the natural taste viewed as adequate and appetizing. Over the last six decades—a relatively short period of time in human digestion history, the gradual reduction in digestible food quality may be why human beings eat more food than ever before.

The creation of engineered ingredients has also allowed for new and advanced food manufacturing methods. These methods employ unique ways to combine overly refined ingredients, thereby extending the shelf life of many recipes. Although cheaper to produce, these new recipes, particularly the ones made with combined chemical additives, ignite cravings and produce taste sensitivities, which encourage overeating.

Recipes engage fat making

From viewing portrait art, it can be assumed secondary fat began accumulating across the human body as early as the fifteenth century. Its birthplace was the kitchens of affluent homes, where multiple-ingredient recipes were being invented. Recipe innovation has continued over the centuries, however, in modern times the use of engineered and chemically created additives has resulted in a digestion counterattack, contributing to many unexpected and incurable biological responses.

Why secondary fat?

Science has not been able to credibly pinpoint why fat accumulates across the entire body. The assumption is, without thorough digestion certain foods and medicines made with indigestible toxins would not be thoroughly digested. These under-digested foods are stored within secondary fat, which would be an automated function, initiated to protect the major organs from toxic exposure.

Secondary fat is not a stationary fat, but a mobile fat, which the digestion distributes without restriction. Whenever the digestion becomes overwhelmed with indigestible ingredients there is a sharp rise in overall body toxicity, particularly when chemically derived hormones and additives accumulate in batches. The digestion's offensive reaction is to store these toxins within secondary fat. The digestion does this as a temporary emergency solution, one employed whenever it is unable to eject toxins from the body using conventional methods.

As a storage mechanism secondary fat is different from body fat, which can be quickly converted into a source of energy. Instead, secondary fat can only be removed after applying specially created and customized enzymes, especially those needed to break down complex toxin profiles.

ഇരു

Factor 1: Enzymes

Enzymes are critical to completing digestion and extracting nutrients. Eating meals, particularly complex-ingredient meals, reduces the time needed to create customized enzymes. This produces inefficient and shortened digestion cycles.

ID - simple enzyme sequence

STAGE ■ Recipes consumed.

STAGE ► Mouth chews; ingredients are sorted; phase 1 enzyme release.

STAGE ► Ingredients are sorted again; chemical additives and hormones are sorted and separated.

STAGE ► Phase 2 enzyme release.

STAGE ► **Disadvantage** - No enzymes on hand to digest complex chemically-created additives.

STAGE ► **Disadvantage** - Immediate secondary fat production and storage.

STAGE ► **Disadvantage** - Secondary fat accumulates in remote areas of the body.

STAGE ► **Disadvantage** - Potential threat of illness after toxin levels rise.

Factor 2: Glucose

In order to turn off secondary fat production and diminish unwanted fat stores, the body must avoid incidents of partial digestion, while at the same time reducing glucose reserves.

The simultaneous manufacturing of two structurally different fats, natural body fat and secondary fat, suggests no individual fat can be efficiently digested when the body is continuously processing new food. In short, the frequency of eating meals, and in a short span of time, interrupts all enzyme distribution cycles, resulting in a constant stream of glucose circulating in the blood. This also suggests glucose is always available, even when nutrients may be less available.

More glucose in circulation.
Not enough nutrients in circulation.

Factor 3: Cravings

When the foods consumed are altered at the molecular level, cravings become more aggressive. In this scenario the desire to eat nutrient deficient foods becomes frequent, particularly if clock eating allows large groupings of molecularly-altered ingredients to gather together during digestion. If these mechanical conflicts happen many times during a single day, people will eat when they are not hungry.

What is natural hunger?

The opposite reaction to cravings is natural hunger. Natural hunger is a physical signaling system used to indicate when the body needs to be nourished. These signals appear as unexpected physical responses, including a general weakness, yawning, or feeling tired. When these prompts happen, this is viewed as a biological request to replenish nutrients.

The fat we eat

The Ingredient Diet does not discourage eating digestible fats. Digestible fats are derived from naturally occurring, single-ingredient, and under-processed foods. These digestible fats are found in simple foods, which have complimentary enzymes, always available to complete digestion cycles. The most compatible fats are found in cleanly derived (naturally produced) meats, eggs, fish, olives, avocados, coconuts, seeds, and nuts. In contrast, the least compatible fats are found in heat-treated, hormone-enhanced, engineered, and synthetically created foods.

Hidden modifications

The molecular modification of any ingredient (at

the cellular level) lowers its digestion value, and as a consequence, handicaps enzyme interactions during digestion. This includes the digestion of fats found in pasteurized dairy.

Pasteurization is a flash heat treatment used to kill potentially unfriendly bacteria. For some people pasteurized milk may be difficult to digest because the molecular structure of the milk has changed. This also suggests augmented milk would be difficult to match with correct enzymes during digestion. A more extensive section on pasteurization can be found on page 180.

Combining recipes

Of all the food categories, because of its sheer density, processed fats interrupt digestion cycles the most, producing what The Ingredient Diet describes as ingredient instability. These conditions are further complicated if the digestion is forced to sort many altered fats (found in different recipes) including combinations of vegetable, olive, corn, and sunflower oils. This is in addition to having to sort various refined sugars such as cane, beet, honey, maple, and agave. This list of ingredients also includes combined grains, meats, and artificially created foods, all melded together. This assembly of complex ingredients would always require special enzyme combinations to complete digestion.

A new diet perspective

The Ingredient Diet introduces a simplification of digestion. This approach requires creating an eating vacuum, or more precisely, allowing digestion to complete each eating cycle. Completing digestion is essential to limiting the production of body fat. However, when there is a stockpile of glucose collected after consuming back to back and sequential meals, fat making would be continuous. These are digestion conditions where reducing fat stores would be difficult. However, if glucose became less available, or quickly exhausted, new fat would be produced less frequently.

Where is fat stored?

The remoteness of secondary fat stores guarantees they will be difficult to access, and as a consequence, difficult to efficiently metabolize. In addition, secondary fat cannot be removed by exercising because it is a storage mechanism for undigested toxins, not a direct source of energy. This fat would first have to undergo a repeated digestion cycle before it could be used as an energy fuel. In addition, because of its toxic composition, secondary fat is structurally complex, making it unstable, unreliable, and difficult to convert into a primary fuel.

Because of these hypothetical digestion conditions, secondary fat removal would always be gradual, particularly when undigested toxins must be located, isolated, and then matched with correct enzymes, before being thoroughly digested.

ഓരു

Digestion final pass

All final digestion efforts require the involvement

of the liver. This is the organ that discharges and helps

eliminate various forms of body waste. The liver also

manufactures, maneuvers, and manipulates fat. Processing

times in the stomach depend on the time needed to digest

complex additives and toxins. For a new additive-rich

meal, the full digestion time would range 18-24 hours.

When large groups of chemically derived

additives, hormones, and preserving agents, cluster

together in the stomach, this assembly of toxic ingredients

causes the digestion process to become unstable. All

under-digested foods and toxins would be quickly

removed to the liver. This initiates the next processing

phase, secondary fat production, which is followed by the transport and storage of fat to remote areas of the body. As secondary fat stores accumulate, this also ensures toxin levels will rise across the body.

ഇരു

The following example describes the hypothetical digestion cycle of a fast food, hamburger and French fries meal. There are multiple ingredients in this meal from those found in the bun, to the meat, mayonnaise, and sauces. This sequence does not include the very involved digestion process used to break down hormones and other preserving ingredients, suggesting completed digestion could take even longer. The estimated time for the complete digestion of this complex meal would range between 18-24 hours. In contrast, a customary (or normal) digestion cycle would take less than eight hours. This includes the time needed to distribute nutrients and eliminate waste.

Observation: As a feature of food evolution, fast foods are no longer classified as restaurant only foods. These overly manufactured foods are now found in almost all grocery store aisles across the world.

Digestion sequence, hamburger and French fries meal

➢Phase 1: The mouth chews the food and introduces the first phase of digestive enzymes.

➢Phase 2: The pre-digested food enters the stomach, and new enzymes begin breaking down the proteins and carbohydrates.

➢Phase 3: The stomach releases more acid enzymes, further breaking down the meat proteins, mayonnaise, and ingredient-rich sauces.

➢Phase 4: Any surplus carbohydrates and sugars (found in the French fries, bun, and sauces) are digested.

➢Phase 5: The digestion begins identifying and sorting the additives, preservatives, and hormones. If any of these ingredients are indigestible, they are removed to the liver for further processing. If the liver becomes overwhelmed with toxins and waste, all undigested toxins are stored as part of secondary fat and remain in the body. This final stage is usually a quick process, intended to move toxins away from the vital organs. Secondary fat then collects in remote areas of the body until better digestion solutions can be discovered. However, these solutions may never be found, particularly if new meals keep arriving, and initiating new digestion cycles.

Digestion counter reactions

When there are a wide range of digestion complications, the effectiveness of pharmaceutical and medical interventions to correct illness and obesity will become less reliable. It will also be next to impossible to discover permanent cures for new illnesses, particularly if the preservatives and hormones in foods keep changing in strength and quantity. These changes are commonplace, and employed by food manufacturers to increase food yields, stockpile foods, and introduce new preserving techniques—all deliberately employed to preserve foods longer.

Reducing body toxicity

The simplest way to reduce body toxicity is to avoid eating overly processed ingredients, recipes, and meals. To prevent further weight gain and illness, this program advocates eating fewer nutritionally vacant and engineered foods, and abandoning many socialized eating behaviors, particularly clock eating, drinking refined alcohols, and eating in the absence of natural hunger.

Review: Key fat removal issues

Secondary fat is not a direct source of energy because it acts as a storage device for indigestible toxins found in engineered, hormone-rich, and preservatives-rich foods. In order to remove secondary fat, all toxins (within the fat) must first be fully digested. Toxin removal may not be immediate, or based on the combination and complexity of toxic elements, might never happen. The removal of secondary fat would also require more time to create the customized enzymes needed to break down complex toxin profiles.

Because the digestion is a self-repairing, organic system, it may be capable of creating most of the unique enzymes it needs. However, when too many complex recipes are eaten during a single meal, this forces the digestion to break down all ingredients at one time, including indigestible toxins. This makes the creation of specialized enzymes less possible, particularly when continuous clock eating prematurely shortens digestion cycles.

Due to their complex structure, processed foods are viewed as toxic and biologically unstable. Any accompanying food additives (chemicals, hormones, or preservatives) would be poorly digested when the unique enzymes needed to digest them are not immediately available.

In all cases, any digestion interruption would shorten the timing of a single digestion window, which is more likely to happen each time a new meal arrives within a 4-6 hour clock eating cycle. These under-digestion events cause toxins to remain in the body, stored as a component of secondary fat. If poor digestion events continue for years and decades, elevated toxin levels will not only result in weight gain, but the possibility of chronic illness exposure when the body reaches its genetically unique toxin threshold.

ID Definitions

Digestion Anxiety or DA – this is digestion exhaustion, which happens when a large influx of processed ingredients forces the digestion to process all ingredients at one time.

Secondary Fat – A new fat-like substance used by the liver to store undigested toxins.

Clock Eating – These are predetermined, socially-conforming food events, encouraging people to eat when they are not hungry.

Recipes – The combining of engineered ingredients to produce new hybrid foods, which trigger taste sensitivities, followed by incomplete digestion.

Tracking Progress
Starts Here!

Please take a moment to record your personal data on one of the trackers found in the Resources section starting on page 257.

Weight Chart for Women

Weight in pounds, based on ages 25–59 with the lowest mortality rate (indoor clothing weighing 5 pounds and shoes with 1-inch heels).

Height in Shoes	Small Frame	Medium Frame	Large Frame
6'	138 to 151	148 to 162	158 to 179
5'11"	135 to 148	145 to 159	155 to 176
5'10"	132 to 145	142 to 156	152 to 173
5'9"	129 to 142	139 to 153	149 to 170
5'8"	126 to 139	136 to 150	146 to 167
5'7"	123 to 136	133 to 147	143 to 163
5'6"	120 to 133	130 to 144	140 to 159
5'5"	117 to 130	127 to 141	137 to 155
5'4"	114 to 127	124 to 138	134 to 151
5'3"	111 to 124	121 to 135	131 to 147
5'2"	108 to 121	118 to 132	128 to 143
5'1"	106 to 118	115 to 129	125 to 140
5'	104 to 115	113 to 126	122 to 137
4'11"	103 to 113	111 to 123	120 to 134
4'10"	102 to 111	109 to 121	118 to 131

From height and weight tables of the Metropolitan Life Insurance Company, 1983.

Weight Chart for Men

Weight in pounds, based on ages 25–59 with the lowest mortality rate (indoor clothing weighing 5 pounds and shoes with 1-inch heels).

Height in Shoes	Small Frame	Medium Frame	Large Frame
6′4″	162 to 176	171 to 187	181 to 207
6′3″	158 to 172	167 to 182	176 to 202
6′2″	155 to 168	164 to 178	172 to 197
6′1″	152 to 164	160 to 174	168 to 192
6′	149 to 160	157 to 170	164 to 188
5′11″	146 to 157	154 to 166	161 to 184
5′10″	144 to 154	151 to 163	158 to 180
5′9″	142 to 151	148 to 160	155 to 176
5′8″	140 to 148	145 to 157	152 to 172
5′7″	138 to 145	142 to 154	149 to 168
5′6″	136 to 142	139 to 151	146 to 164
5′5″	134 to 140	137 to 148	144 to 160
5′4″	132 to 138	135 to 145	142 to 156
5′3″	130 to 136	133 to 143	140 to 153
5′2″	128 to 134	131 to 141	138 to 150

From height and weight tables of the Metropolitan Life Insurance Company, 1983.

Chapter 5

Meals v Windows

> ಇಿಂಚ
> "Take away food from a sick man's stomach and you have begun, not to starve the sick man, but the disease."
> —E. H. Dewey, M.D.

By choice, not design

Historically, the human biology has proved adaptive in times of famine, food sacrifice, and scarcity. Essential to their beliefs, Muslims, Catholics, Orthodox Jews, and Buddhist monks, participate in various forms of food abstinence. Even prisoners of war have survived long periods of exile without eating regular meals. This last example would be the most severe, but like the others

93

illustrates the body's resilience and adaptability when no solid foods are eaten for longer durations of time.

Being obsessed about when to eat breakfast, lunch, and dinner—or how to manage foods as part of a special diet, or even selecting the tastiest dessert—all of these decisions add stress to the organic digestion process. Also, whenever the body doesn't get food it doesn't immediately shut down, instead it uses its stored reserves of fat to manage its energy needs. Unless illness requires eating food regularly, the majority of us can do without eating timed meals.

Body maintenance

Avoiding set meal schedules could also be viewed as opportunities when the body resets to improve physical performance. This form of **closed window** offers the digestion a break from digesting solid foods. These are also times when the body restores enzyme systems, almost like a mini vacation. Most of us take vacations, so why shouldn't our digestion get one as well?

94

Why diets don't work

Certain weight management programs encourage eating high quality and easily digestible ingredients, at the same time isolating foods to permanently avoid. These systems not only help the dieter reduce excess body fat and lose weight, but uncover (and permanently avoid) specific indigestible foods.

In contrast, other diets conform to clock eating by introducing meal-focused menus, and encouraging dieters to eat multiple-ingredient foods. These plans are presented as short term endeavors, allowing old eating behaviors to resume once the diet ends. These diets also encourage counting calories, reducing fatty foods, using cleanses and shakes, or eating protein exclusively. Theoretically, all of these strategies are designed to initiate fat loss, however, all of these strategies also streamline and avoid certain ingredients. Coincidentally, many of these diets require avoiding foods made with heat treated fats and refined sugars. This is followed by the unexpected and perhaps unnoticed benefit of gradually reducing body toxicity as the digestion process becomes increasingly more efficient.

Can I stick with this diet?

Modern diets have also made popular programs incorporating overly processed foods, frozen meals, bars, and shakes; as well as the most debilitating of all dieting concepts, consuming more animal protein than the body can properly digest. Offering one respected form of food control, juice cleanses have been used to rejuvenate health. When administered with nutrition in mind, this particular method can calm the digestion by strategically eliminating solid foods.

Similar to other digestion-focused methods, The Ingredient Diet emphasizes the importance of eating fresh, nutrient-dense, single ingredient foods, at the same time avoiding overly processed, refined, engineered, heat-treated, and pasteurized foods.

Avoiding clock eating

Cleansing programs are a form of **closed window,** or extended times without eating solid food. These fast acting, short term protocols produce a more alert digestion, at the same time efficiently distributing nutrients across the body.

In contrast, social and robotic eating behaviors infer that going without solid food is unacceptable; and because of busy work and life schedules we find large segments of the population eating at routine times of the day, even when their bodies are not requesting nutrition. Automated meal schedules also represent times when it is convenient to eat, suggesting meals have become a series of daily tasks, and not nutrition replenishment activities.

Meals with identities

Why has breakfast been labeled the most important meal of the day, and who created this label? This is particularly curious when the complexity and largess of ingredients consumed during the dinner meal may not have completed digestion by the time the person arises from slumber. In this scenario breakfast would not be the most important meal of the day, but the least necessary meal of the day. Eating breakfast when the digestion is still processing a previous meal is a robotic eating behavior, and often promoted by social programming, prescription drug requirements, commercial diets, and food industry advertising.

80Q3

Meal tags

The tagging of implied meal associations also sells nutritionally-vacant recipes. For example, many recipes are labeled breakfast foods, including cereals, pancakes, waffles, and breakfast bars. In reality these foods have no special designations and could be eaten at any time. This is particularly curious when the digestion, being a simple organism, would not be able to distinguish socially labeled foods.

In contrast, without these designations the only reason to eat food would be to increase energy and boost nutrition. Replacing these conditioned eating behaviors would also simplify many food-related tasks, limit unnecessary cooking, grocery shopping, meal planning, and managing different recipes at social events.

Eliminating meals

Prior to the twentieth century eating one meal a day, supper, was the common practice. This meal was usually eaten early evening, often before sunset. Eating fewer meals may sound difficult, even controversial, however, it is far removed from present day eating behaviors. In fact, prior to the Victorian era humans had survived centuries without a formal eating plan.

It's OK to avoid meals...Really it is!

The Ingredient Diet advocates avoiding conventional meal times and eating fewer poor-quality ingredients. This would involve introducing a new eating schedule, one focused on improving digestion efficiency. This strategy also encourages eating only when there is true hunger, or when the body needs or asks for nutrition.

There are digestion benefits associated with avoiding set meal times. The most significant improvement would be installing a supportive system of ingredient reduction. This reduction system would compliment lifestyle routines, but at the same time provide sufficient nourishment to support a highly functioning mind and body. Understandably, it may be difficult giving up scheduled meals, particularly for those who are overweight or obese, where meals have become part of a daily to-do list, dictated by commercial diets and social programming.

Introducing the ID strategy

The Ingredient Diet also encourages creating a digestion environment, which allows for consistent fat loss. As described in previous chapters, when the digestion is efficient, the body will naturally employ a

100

heightened repair mode, one that speeds up digestion, at the same time removing excess secondary fat, body fat, and accumulated toxins.

In contrast, when a person engages in clock eating, digestion is constantly being interrupted. This is in addition to being preoccupied managing elevated blood sugar levels, removing toxins, and activating the most undesirable of all biological defensive strategies, storing new and larger reserves of fat. These digestion disruptions also hinder nutrition extraction, which may eventually contribute to unexpected illnesses, both great and small.

ℰ⒨ℛ

The ID strategy

The following ID eating strategy is 100 percent customizable, with no special recipes, processed foods, or calorie-counting requirements. This strategy helps to simplify dietary selection and eating frequency, while focusing on one goal, improving digestion performance.

This strategy also

➢ naturally removes excess secondary fat;

➢ improves wellness markers including mental clarity;

➢ speeds up digestion, thereby enhancing more efficient enzyme utilization;

➢ removes complex ingredients and recipes from the overall diet;

➢ introduces designated times without eating solid food, which improves overall digestion efficiency.

Windows

Clock eating is replaced by **window eating**. This does not require fasting or using cleanses because the eating windows deliberately open and close to accept nutrition. The period of time without food (the **closed window**) can be adjusted. However, the closed window must be long enough to ensure completed digestion.

The closed window can also be extended anywhere between twelve to seventeen hours. The extended time without solid food allows the body to efficiently distribute nutrients to the cells, muscles, organs, and skeleton. These are also times when the digestion is not processing any new food.

The open window—changing digestion rhythms

When it comes to installing a new eating protocol, the first challenge is to create a customized plan to compliment *your* body's nutritional needs. Customized eating allows the body to decide if and when a nutrition boost is needed. When the eating window opens, the body may or may not be asking for nutrition—and the question to ask is, does the body need solid food the moment the eating window opens?

To monitor results, tracking tools have been added to the Resources section of this book. A medical doctor or nutritionist can also offer more guidance as to how to manage a nutrition-focused eating schedule. Keep in mind, eating windows are designed to improve overall digestion, not avoid food.

A single eating window also allows for the monitoring of ingredients. This window is not focused on weight loss, but replenishing nutrients and allowing the various body systems greater access to these nutrients.

The closed window

The **closed window** is a specific time when the body does not receive solid food. These are times when the digestion rebuilds its enzyme reserves, as it anticipates and prepares for the next batch of food to arrive. Although no solid foods are eaten, single ingredient beverages are allowed, including coffee, organic coconut water, and herbal teas.

It is important that the body is always well nourished, and this requires the closed window to reopen. The closed window should not exceed twelve to seventeen hours, and when the eating window reopens, the body receives adequate amounts of high-quality nutrition. The closed windows should be a regular daily event, a minimum of three hundred days a year. This allows for an annual surplus of **I-Free** days, which can be used for random social engagements, holidays, vacations, and parties. More about I-Free days in Chapter Six.

ℰℭ

Ingredient-timing example

The Ingredient Diet reduction programs are described in more detail in Chapters 6 and 7. The following window timing examples are for illustration purposes only.

1:00 p.m. to 8:00 p.m.—Open Window (eating allowed)

- No more than thirty ingredients (ID1 plan) are eaten during the open window. See Chapter 7.

- Single ingredients and limited-ingredient recipes are consumed during the open window.

- High-quality ingredients are consumed, including fruits, vegetables, meats, fish, and cleanly-derived fats, as well as unprocessed and under processed ingredients—and as much as possible, foods created without additives, chemicals, or hormones.

- There are no quantity restrictions, but there is a high nutrition focus for all ingredients consumed during the open window.

ಐ ೮ಶ

8:00 p.m. to 1:00 p.m.— Closed Window

- No solid foods are eaten during the closed window, allowing for more time to complete digestion and distribute nutrients.

ಐ ೮ಶ

Closed window benefits

➢ Offers rest and balance for all body systems as part of a daily recalibration process.

➢ Stops the buildup of unnecessary and surplus fat stores.

➢ Reduces and eliminates accumulated body toxins.

➢ Improves enzyme delivery systems, allowing for more efficient digestion.

Note: For those carrying excess body fat, consuming sugary foods and complex-ingredient meals would not be needed for energy. Existing natural fat reserves would be used for this purpose.

ID Calories

An ID food choice is one that offers the body easily digestible calories. These are nutrient-rich calories, which the digestion easily recognizes, and can quickly and efficiently break down. These calories should come from digestion-friendly, identifiable, and single ingredient foods. Examples include vegetables, fruit, high-quality fats, and proteins.

Because many dieters may already be overweight or even obese, calorie control without definition could lead to cravings, which would be followed by unanticipated overeating. Under these conditions the body accumulates unwanted fat, particularly if many

engineered and processed ingredients remain under-

digested. Not unusual, these are also circumstances where

cravings and the desire to eat more food would intensify.

> **The simplest and most often used measure of abdominal obesity is waist size. Guidelines generally define abdominal obesity in women as a waist size 35 inches or higher, and in men as a waist size of 40 inches or higher.**
>
> *Harvard School of Public Health - See Reference.*

Why avoid meals?

As already discussed, eating meals at customary

mealtimes is a societal behavioral response. Although we

must eat to sustain life, using a predetermined eating

schedule is not needed to meet survival objectives. Eating

breakfast because it is morning, lunch because noon has

arrived, and dinner because it is the last meal before going

to bed, are of little consequence to an organism that does

not recognize socially labeled schedules. Instead, these are

behaviors imposed by business requirements, cultural

beliefs, popular diets, medical ideologies, and unrestricted food marketing.

Ingredient management

Chapter Seven introduces The Ingredient Guidelines. These guidelines have been designed to avoid episodes of digestion anxiety. The overall intention is to increase and deliver more nutrients during digestion.

Ingredient monitoring involves

➢ introducing the dieter to new ingredient selection rituals, further isolating how, what, and when foods are eaten;

➢ eliminating food additives, preservatives, and hormones, to ensure completed digestion;

➢ noticing, avoiding, and tracking cravings;

➢ allowing for the natural and gradual depletion of secondary fat deposits, particularly fat accumulation in various remote areas of the body (arms, belly, lower extremities, face, and neck);

➢ retraining the taste buds and sensory taste mechanism to crave more nutritious foods. Foods, which in the past may have been viewed as less tasty. This nutrition retraining also discourages cravings for salt, sugars, and chemically derived sweeteners;

➢ reducing blood acidity by managing pH. This potentially discourages future threats of illness and chronic disease. More about pH in Chapter 8.

Review: Window approach

By following the ID window strategy the body adjusts to eating fewer ingredients, eating more nutritious foods, and eating less often.

When the eating window opens, consuming single-ingredient and nutrient dense foods restricts poor-quality ingredients, at the same time improving digestion efficiency, and avoiding incidents of new fat storage. Although the **open window** does not adhere to limiting any food category—fats, carbohydrates, and proteins are allowed, multiple ingredient combinations (or complicated recipes) are restricted. This program also grants the digestion uninterrupted access to secondary fat stores, allowing for the removal of all fat types, which as an additional benefit reduces unwanted toxins.

ಬಿಂಐಎಸ್

ID Definitions

OPEN (EATING) WINDOW—A time when the digestion is highly responsive, active, and flushed with enzyme reserves.

CLOSED (EATING) WINDOW – A time when the body distributes nutrition to revitalize the cells, boost dietary enzymes, and deplete fat stores. No solid foods are consumed during the closed window.

ID10 – A strategy for counting and managing ingredients. ▶ID10 gradually reduces the quantity of ingredients eaten. ▶ID10 is used to isolate and identify ingredients in recipes and multiple ingredient meals. ▶ID10 avoids unknown additives, which cannot be counted accurately.

I-FREE DAYS - No ingredient counting. Extra days to participate in food events and social gatherings.

NID = Non ID. These are severely restricted foods.

"An increasing number of animal studies have shown altered markers for health in subjects exposed to intermittent fasting, i.e. regularly and repeatedly abstaining from eating during 12-36 hours per period. It has been hypothesized that the reported beneficial health effects from caloric restriction on excess body weight, cardiovascular risk factors, glucose metabolism, tumor physiology, neurodegenerative pathology and life span, can be mimicked by alternating periods of short term fasting with periods of refeeding, without deliberately altering the total caloric intake. Therefore, a systematic review of available intervention studies on intermittent fasting and animal and human health was performed. In rodents, intermittent fasting exhibits beneficial effects, including decreased body weight, improved cardiovascular health and glucose regulation, enhanced neuronal health, decreased cancer risk and increased life span – some of the effects independent of the effects attributed to calorie restriction alone. The human studies performed to date are generally of low-quality design. Beneficial effects such as weight loss, reduced risk for cardiovascular disease and improved insulin sensitivity have been observed, but conflicting data exists."

—Dr. Bojan Kostevski; http://www.lift-heavy.com

Chapter 6

The ID Plans + Ingredients

⎧ **Chapter 6 and 7 introduce the** ⎫
⎩ **ingredient identification method.** ⎭

Limiting meals—it's not hard!

Diets created in the last two decades have been designed to maneuver through social interactions, which has created a dependence on eating at specific times. The Ingredient Diet is designed to change these behaviors by interrupting, removing, and replacing meals, at the same time managing cravings, and providing the body with more digestible nutrition. Most of these cravings are often triggered by cultural and social responses to food, and make irresistible many allergy-causing ingredients, overly refined ingredients, fast foods, and meals eaten at predetermined times of the day.

The ID plans presented next, focus on reducing and removing poor quality ingredients and improving overall digestion performance. These systems are designed to deliver more high-quality and easily digestible nutrition to the entire body, while allowing enough time to remove toxins, rid the body of secondary fat, and minimize cravings.

By installing digestion cycles versus meals, both ID plans boost nutrition. That said, it is important to restate the purpose of these plans, which is to replace indigestible foods with nutrient-dense foods.

Plan introduction

Over the centuries, and as part of numerous social eating practices (religious, health, strife, and environmental) people have used different approaches to stagger food intake. Eating windows offer a similar method of streamlining foods, while at the same time reducing indigestible ingredients in the overall diet. Both

ID plans further discourage a dependency on socially

ordained meals.

The **ID1** plan introduces a timing strategy that

deliberately reduces and eliminates indigestible

ingredients. In contrast, **ID2** is not timing specific,

allowing for a larger (but modest) number of ingredients.

Each plan can be used independently, for example,

starting with ID2, and then easing into ID1. This allows

for a gradual reduction in ingredients, while allowing the

digestion to remove fat and improve nutrient distribution

across the body. If used as a weight loss program, these

plans can be adjusted, for example, six weeks on ID1,

followed by 6 weeks on ID2. They can also be used as a

lifetime eating approach, used to bolster natural immunity.

Beyond the importance of increasing absorbable

nutrients, both plans emphasize the importance of

identifying cravings, particularly if giving in to cravings

may be one reason why a diet fails. The Ingredient Diet is

not a calorie reduction plan, but a deliberate way to

increase nutrient absorption, while at the same time

avoiding any digestion interruptions, which initiate fat

making.

Interrupting fat production

If both fat production and reducing body fat are

dependent on insulin delivery systems, then understanding

insulin overproduction can improve dieting outcomes. If

food rituals involve eating too many overly processed

ingredients, including refined sugars and carbohydrates,

and when these rituals are enjoyed for years and decades,

insulin production will remain in overproduction. This

type of unmonitored food consumption shifts customary

fat production into overdrive.

Fat production on overdrive

In situations where the overall diet is filled with

refined ingredients, including heat-treated oils, starches,

and processed sugars, all being digested at one time, the

blood chemistry will always be flooded with blood sugar.

All this digestion debris must go somewhere, and that somewhere is fat production. Using an extended closed window (no solid foods eaten for a longer period of time) encourages the digestion to properly utilize enzymes and thoroughly digest all foods. This also allows nutrition to be quickly extracted and distributed, resulting in less digestion debris and glucose remaining in the blood.

Readiness

Both ID plans are contrary to how we socially eat. However, in a world where regular meal cycles are expected, eating using a minimizing approach may possibly symbolize deprivation—when this is not the case at all. This does not mean avoid food, friends, or social situations, but instead engage in digestion-focused eating, especially in situations where ingredient counting may be unpredictable.

80 03

The ID plans have been designed to not only support completed digestion, but also accommodate the dieter's lifestyle. Although the ID1 window replaces clock eating, this is not considered fasting because all windows open and close each day. The window without food, the **closed window**, can be customized longer or shorter, and can last as long as twelve to seventeen hours. Finally, adopting new eating times may produce unexpected physical responses, including headaches, migraines, blurry vision, nausea, and feelings of anxiousness. However, these reactions would be normal and temporary, particularly when the body is adjusting to a more relevant schedule of nutrition delivery.

ID Program Note: The following windows and plans may not be suitable for those with severe health issues or suffer from blood sugar imbalances regulated by medication. Before starting, seek the advice of a medical professional.

Windows

The Open and Closed windows are used in conjunction with the ID plans. These are not fasting plans, but longer times without eating complex recipes and ingredient-rich meals. These windows can also be customized to fit the individual's lifestyle. By combining windows and plans over multiple and consecutive six-week cycles, weight-loss and health goals become more achievable. This is followed by ID3, which ensures ingredient management becomes a lifetime, must-do activity.

ID1- The Concentrated Reduction Plan

I.   ID1 includes up to 30 (nutrient-dense) ingredients, eaten during the open window.

II. ID1 limits multiple ingredients using the ID10 approach (see page 123).

III. ID1 encourages eating enough high-quality and nutrient-dense foods during the open window.

For ID1 all windows can be adjusted longer or shorter.

This ensures twelve to seventeen hours without eating

solid food called the **closed window**. The closed window is timed to incorporate the hours spent sleeping, which helps to curb some of the physical and emotional discomfort experienced in the early stages of the plan, when the dieter is attempting to avoid high ingredient meals.

ID1—the open window, how does it work?

For ID1, after the eating window opens, there can be as many as three ID10 eating events. These add up to thirty consumed ingredients during the open window. To manage this process it is important to accurately count all ingredients consumed. It is also important to eat only when the body is asking for food, or offers a signal of natural hunger. ID1 encourages eating during a shorter window of time, and more important, to eat only when the digestion is alert, responsive, and able to accept a new batch of food.

ID10

The **ID10** concept was created after researching classic recipes made with fewer ingredients. ID10 requires eating ten or fewer ingredients at one time. These ten (or fewer) ingredients are eaten during the open window, can be grouped together, or can be combined as part of simple recipes. These smaller ingredient groupings should not include foods created with hormones, pesticides, and additives.

ID2 - the Consistent Reduction Plan

I.ID2 includes 30-50 (nutrient-dense) ingredients per day.

II. ID2 does not use windows.

ID2 is ingredient-generous, and designed to reduce ingredient counts while offering more lifestyle flexibility. ID2 introduces an ingredient management approach focused on improving food quality and nutrient absorption. More about ID2 in Chapter 7.

ID3—Maintenance

Ingredient counts are the same for ID2 and ID3, except ID3 is a maintenance strategy where ingredient counting and selection become a way of life. Maintenance is introduced after weight loss objectives have been reached on ID1, the dieter becomes more familiar with ingredient counting, and the dieter can easily recognize those foods their body cannot easily digest.

I-Free Day

The I-Free day is free of windows and ingredient restrictions. These allow for social eating, and food occasions where ingredient counting may be difficult.

ഇരു

Open window—how long should it stay open?

Overall, the goal of the open window is to optimize enzyme performance. The open window can last as long as ten hours, and eating is staggered across this time. All consumed ingredients are naturally derived and easily countable. By staggering and consuming fewer ingredients, this ensures all foods are thoroughly digested, and all digestion cycles complete quickly and efficiently.

ಬಿ ೮ಠ

ID1 Example:

The eating window opens at 1pm. The first consumed ingredient is an unripe (not overripe) banana. The dieter than waits one hour for digestion to finalize before eating again.

> *Unripe fruit has less sugar, which allows enzymes to digest the fiber and nutrition without interruptions. This also helps avoid any sharp spikes in blood sugar.*

The next serving of ingredients (at 2 pm) includes a small quantity of cleanly produced nuts. This can be followed with a salad made with non-starch vegetables, adding avocado and lemon dressing. Dieters always select ingredients they can easily count. This style of ingredient selection continues until the window closes at 8PM. The total number of ingredients consumed during the open window is 30 (ID1 plan limit).

Black coffee, organic coconut water, and teas, are permitted without restrictions, and these are counted as free ingredients. All forms of added sugar and dairy are avoided.

›‹

ID1 for weight loss

As with most diets, the starting point requires setting a goal. The next step is weighing in, which provides a benchmark for tracking future weight loss and

126

fat loss.

Another supportive measuring tool is using a blood-monitoring device (optional). This tracks improvements in blood sugar. Blood sugar measurements are taken at the end of the closed window, when the digestion is less active. On ID1, after two, six-week cycles, blood sugar and weight loss are measured again, and this is followed by a new 6-week cycle. These six-week cycles allow enough time for the blood to recycle and remove toxins.

The first six week cycle

- Before beginning any aspect of this strategy, consult with a doctor to determine whether this program is suitable for current health circumstances and lifestyle.
- Weight loss is measured on day one of ID1, and again on the last day of week six. To help monitor results, tracking tools have been added to the Resources section.
- For additional tracking, blood sugar can be

monitored and measured. The first screening is taken on day one, and repeated on the last day of week six.

- I-Free and eating windows can be customized to fit the individual's lifestyle and routines. The ID plans are not fasting programs, but longer times without eating ingredient-rich recipes and meals.

- To further streamline ingredients, ID10 groupings are used to limit ingredients to 10 or fewer, which further restricts preservatives and processed additives.

- Eating resumes when the eating window reopens, and for **no more than ten hours**. <u>This is the maximum time the eating window is open every day.</u> The eating window opens when the body is alert, active, and asking for a nutrition boost.

- To avoid emotional stress, single-ingredient fluids (unlimited quantities) are allowed during the closed window. Under-processed, lower-acidity coffee, organic coconut water, and herbal teas, are allowed all day. No dairy allowed. No juices allowed. No added sugar or sweeteners allowed (except Stevia). For improved health, generational grains are best avoided or eliminated.

ಬಿ ಛ

The four ID rules
Rule 1—Tracking

Locate your individual weight range on the height and weight charts provided on page 89. Weigh and record your beginning body weight using one of the tracking tools found in the Resources section.

Rule 2—Window times

Consistent window timing improves digestion efficiency. For ID1, once the times have been selected for the open and closed windows, stick to these times for the entire six week cycle. The most adaptable open window begins at 1:00 p.m. Using the previous example, solid foods are not consumed between 8:00 p.m. and 1:00 p.m., or seventeen hours without solid food. The window then reopens between 1:00 p.m. and 8:00 p.m. During the open cycle the dieter selects foods from The Ingredient Guide (see Chapter Seven). The primary goal is to eat more nutritious foods. This is not a time to overeat, but a time to focus on digestion efficiency and nutrition replenishment.

The next goal is to manage the closed window. This means no solid foods are eaten after the window closes. This is the longest period without food, allowing more time to digest all foods, while accessing and depleting secondary fat stores across the body.

	Window Closed	Window Opens
Day 1-6	8:00 PM - 1:00 PM	1:00 PM to 8:00 PM
Day 7	Random ingredients allowed.	
I-Free Day (IFD)	IFD is explained in more detail later.	

Illustration 2: Window Eating Example

ႸჂ Ⴚჵ

Rule 3—Limited exercise - at least initially!

It is recommended that no vigorous exercise be conducted during the first six-week cycle. This allows the digestion to adjust to a new eating schedule.

Rule 4—Read these rules again

Diets often fail because the dieter forgets their wellness objectives. Reading the first three rules once a week can help maintain dieting momentum.

ଚ୍ଚ ଔ

How to eat during the open window

The eating window opens for a specific time—example, seven hours. Based on the plan chosen, the dieter eats reasonable amounts of ingredients, chosen from the Ingredient Guidelines (see next chapter). When the window closes, approximately eight (or more) of the seventeen hours are spent sleeping. Closed windows are not viewed as fasting because unsweetened, single-ingredient coffees, organic coconut water, and teas, are

131

allowed.

Eat enough food

During the open window calorie counting is helpful—not for restricting eating, but for making sure sufficient calories are being consumed. The body must receive an adequate amount of food to extract a sufficient amount of nutrition. The standard calorie count for most commercial diets is between 1200 and 1800 calories a day, however, more calories can be added depending on the frequency and intensity of exercise, (see program rules).

It is important to eat enough high-quality and nutrient-dense ingredients when the eating window opens. This encourages satiation, avoids cravings, and adds more digestible nutrients to the overall diet.

The mind is in charge

As a reminder, meals such as breakfast, lunch, and dinner, are societal concepts, not eating patterns the organic digestion understands. The foremost digestion villain is the meal called dinner, which is often the largest ingredient-saturated meal of the day. In modern times dinner is usually eaten after sunset, when the body tends to be less active and the digestion is slower.

In the early stages of the plan, when cravings are the strongest, the desire to eat poor-quality and nutrient-vacant foods may be difficult to resist. Keeping busy and focused, particularly during the closed window, can help manage these new eating routines.

⁝⁞

ID2—The Flexible Plan

➤ The purpose of ID2 is to reduce and manage ingredients to improve long-range health.

➤ ID2 allows 30-50 nutrient dense ingredients per day, eaten at any time (no closed window).

➤ Limited or **no** preserving ingredients allowed.

➤ **NO** additives or engineered foods.

➤ Blood testing is optional.

➤If economically feasible, all solid foods should be of the highest quality nutrition, in-season fruits and vegetables, and have low ingredient scores. See the Ingredient Counting and Scoring Guidelines in Chapter 7.

I-Free Days (IFD)

➤ I-Free days allow for social eating. However, these are not go-crazy days, where the dieter eats uncontrollable amounts of multiple-ingredient foods and combined recipes.

➤ Flexibility supports five to six days on ID1 or ID2, and then one or two I-Free days (if necessary).

ID Bonus Ingredients

Approved beverages include purely derived water, espresso coffee, organic coconut water, and teas.

- Espresso coffee is preferred because it has a lower acidity than most conventionally brewed coffees. Pay attention to excess caffeine, which can trigger cravings.

- Herbal teas have less caffeine. Kombucha tea is a fermented tea known to have digestion benefits.

- Coconut water (organic preferred) offers the body minerals and electrolytes. With its lower sugar values, it can also be used to replace fruit juices.

Review: Part 1 - Windows

The open and closed windows encourage eating fewer ingredients, complex meals, and unnecessary snacks. This would be a departure from the newest of all dietary trends, eating meals made with many indigestible recipes and large quantities of engineered proteins.

These windows also serve to identify cravings, particularly cravings, which ignore the body's legitimate requests for nutrition. When the body is well-nourished, the need to overeat or crave unhealthy foods will lessen over time.

ഇൗ൪

Review: Part 2 - ID Plans
ID1—The window plan

➢ ID1 allows eating thirty (30) high quality ingredients per day. These ingredients are eaten during a timed window of eating called the Open Window.

➢ Limited or **no** preserving ingredients allowed.

➢ **NO** additives or engineered foods.

➢ This counting strategy relies on eating solid foods during a set period of time.

➢ When the eating window opens, eating and ingredient counting begin at the same time. When the window closes, no solid foods are eaten, allowing the digestion to process with minimal interruptions until the window reopens.

136

➤ Window times are customizable. As a general rule, the window time chosen should include the hours spent sleeping, plus an additional 8-10 hours without consuming solid food.

➤ The longer the window remains closed (no solid foods are consumed) the body is focused on digesting and removing stored fat.

➤ The closed window should be a consistent time every day, which allows the body to adjust to a new and accelerated nutrient delivery schedule.

ℬℭ

EASY BEGINNER STEPS

Step One:

This applies to both ID Plans.

a. Pick a monitoring tool from the Resources section.

b. Weigh in and record your personal goals (both weight loss and health).

See weight charts on page 89.

Step Two:

D. Select your personal open and closed window times. These windows will be used consistently for the next six weeks and beyond. Choose times easily fitting your schedule and lifestyle.

Step Three:

E. Record and score the ingredients consumed every day (including additives). This is critical to managing weight loss.

Step Four:

F. Weigh in and record your weight every 6 weeks.

Step Five:

G. Allow for no more than one I-Free day per week during the first 6-week cycle.

Chapter 7

Counting Ingredients

> **DEFINITION OF ENGINEERED FOOD**
>
> Any food created using artificial means,
> which includes preservatives, pesticides,
> pasteurization, heat processing,
> fertilizers, genetic modifications,
> chemical enhancements, additives, and
> hormones.

Ingredient scoring

How many ingredients do you suppose you eat every day? How many ingredients in just one meal? Sometimes there are too many ingredients to count, and many more ingredients when different foods and recipes are prepared in different ways. Another not so obvious factor, one that indirectly affects digestion quality, how many chemicals and hormones (in individual ingredients) are used to create the foods we enjoy eating? This includes the many pesticides used to grow potatoes, and the hormones fed to a single cow. Keep in mind, these are the same ingredients used to create a future hamburger and French fries meal.

 හ ශ

Remember, whatever feeds food will feed you, too.

Ingredient interactions

It would be a pure guess just how many ingredients people consume, as many as 1,000 to 1,500 ingredients weekly, and perhaps even more ingredients after cravings have been triggered.

Equally uncertain, little research is available to explain how engineered and processed ingredients interact during digestion, or how these interactions impact nutrient absorption. Offering one example, **if a food governing agency approves a single synthetic additive for manufacturing or agricultural use, it is highly likely that at some point during digestion this additive will touch, combine, converge, or incorporate with many other approved, chemically-created additives. These are the interactions which cause harm to the human body.**[6]

ঃ৩ ৫৪

---

[6] See Plate Diagram on page 20.

Reduction process

The Ingredient Diet strategy is designed to avoid adverse ingredient interactions. This diet is not focused on portion or calorie control, but ingredient control, coupled with natural digestion efficiency.

Reducing poor ingredient interactions requires paying close attention to every ingredient eaten, and avoiding recipes prepared with multiple ingredients and complex additives. The following guidelines, as well as pH management discussed in Chapter 8, can be used to qualify ingredients. These guidelines can be used with the ID1 and ID2 plans to improve and accelerate digestion efficiency, promote consistent weight loss, boost nutrition, support disease-free health, and strengthen the immunity.

80 03

Ingredient strategy

1. All ID plans avoid or limit overly processed fats, sugars, grains, and additives.

2. The recipes consumed should have obvious and countable ingredients.

3. The daily maximum for ID1 is 30 ingredients, *excluding* free ingredients.

4. The daily maximum for ID2 is up to 50 ingredients, *excluding* free ingredients.

5. Both plans avoid additives, hormones, preservatives, pesticides, fillers, and unknown ingredients.

6. Ingredient monitoring is used to manage and reduce overall ingredients.*

*Monitoring tools have been included in the Resources section.

Social ingredients

Due to our human need to socialize, it is next to impossible to ignore social interactions or avoid events with ingredient-rich foods. In modern times the strongest reactions to cravings could easily be ignited during familiar events such as family gatherings, social interactions, and holidays. For example, food triggers or eating favorite foods such as birthday cake, pecan pie, and honey-baked ham, have sentimental appeal and are automatically linked to certain festivities. However, these classic recipes and many other foods, are not of the same molecular construction today as they were when first enjoyed. The ingredients used to make them have changed, and in many situations (if not all) these sentimental recipes are now constructed with highly refined or engineered ingredients, which at some point in their development may have been exposed to hormones, pesticides, and fertilizers. Not only do these foods taste different today, they will taste different next year, and year after year, because the ingredients and associated recipes keep changing.

଼ଉ ଓଃ

Ingredient Selection Guide

Basic counting and scoring premise

1. Most ID foods count as 1 ingredient. The following are exceptions to the rule and Non-ID ingredients (**NIDs**). These ingredients require additional time to digest because they produce higher toxicity both during and after digestion. **NIDs should be avoided.**

2. When there is an eating event, there may be many instances of milk or other dairy, as well as various meat choices. Each category has a single ingredient count, one for the total dairy, and one for the total meat. This is because the enzymes needed to break down both of these foods (meat or dairy) will differ, but all foods in the same category (example dairy) may use similar enzymes during a single digestion cycle.

Ingredient Avoid List*	
• Soy (unless non GMO) • All generational grains, (see page 195) including gluten-free. • Non-organic alcohols (avoid)	• Pasteurized dairy (limit) • Heat-treated oils (avoid) • Nonorganic eggs (free range preferred/always natural feed) • Sugars (all) (AVOID)

Illustration 3:Avoid Foods

Counting and Scoring (continued)

Dairy

> = 1 count - raw milk (less common)

> = 2 count - pasteurized milk (more common)

Almost all modern dairy is pasteurized. Pasteurization alters foods at the molecular level, making these foods difficult to match with enzymes. This type of molecular alteration ensures there will be processing delays during digestion. These delays are extended when the dairy is eaten with other non-dairy foods, meats, grains, and sugars. Any interrupted enzyme activity will shorten a digestion cycle, this includes shorter times for nutrient extraction and distribution. When viewed as a form of food alteration, the digestion would always isolate pasteurized foods as being an unreliable source of nutrition.

Non-starch vegetables (combined or eaten alone)

> = Free (examples include lettuce, tomatoes, kale, onions, and many others)

Starchy and root vegetables*

> = 2 count

*Most starchy and root vegetables trigger surplus blood sugar during digestion. Because these are

146

nutrient-dense and fibrous, they are not excluded foods, but should be limited. Examples include potatoes, sweet potatoes, and yams.

Counting Example 1

Meat(1) + dairy(2) + tomatoes(free) + potatoes(2) = Total 5. Add processed butter (or oil) and salt to the potato, 5+5+5 = Total 15. This total does not include hormones and additives, which would not be obvious, and could not be counted accurately.

ဆာ ၺ

Fruit: The Complex Ingredient

Fresh fruit, when not combined with other foods, digest quickly, offering the body fructose, nutrients, and fiber. Preferred varieties of fruit have a higher alkaline pH value (See Chapter 8 for pH guidelines).

Because unripe fruit and non-starchy vegetables are free ingredients, these count as "all you can eat." Dried fruit would be excluded because they are usually overripe, and in some way preserved to extend their packaging shelf life.

Digesting quickly, fructose can slow down the digestion of other foods it combines with, particularly proteins, carbohydrates, and fats. When this happens, all nutrients would be poorly extracted and distributed.

Do not waste ingredient quotas eating overripe fruit.

Counting Fruit

= Free if fruit is under ripe and alkaline forming (see Chapter 8).

Example: An under ripe banana would be semi-hard and light green in color.

= 2 count per ripe fruit

Example: Light yellow banana.

= 5 count per over ripe fruit.

Example: Dark yellow with brown spots indicate the banana is overripe. Ripe bananas have a higher sugar content, and after being consumed, cause blood glucose levels to sharply rise and fat production to begin.

Fruit Tip 1: Because fruit digests quickly, allow one to two hours after eating fresh fruit for digestion to complete before eating any other food categories.

Fruit TIP 2: Always eat fruits in season and grown in your geographical area. The following produce guide (link) can be useful for identifying seasonal fruits.

148

When focusing specifically on the digestion of fruit, the availability of enzymes also depends on factors such as geography and climate changes. For more about fruit management see page 230.

http://www.sustainabletable.org/seasonalfoodguide/

Fruit Juice Combinations

= 5 count per juice.

For shakes and smoothies counting depends on what type of fruit, and how many different juices are selected for one drink. Because the fiber has been removed, drinking fruit juice alone *does not* have the same benefits as eating whole, fresh, and under ripe fruit. Fruit juices break down quickly into fructose (fruit sugars). Depending on the pace of digestion, juices may not be a stable source of energy or nutrients. A preferred juice alternative is organic coconut water.

Dieters who suffer from low blood sugar and regularly drink fruit juice, should consult with their physician before beginning this program.

Non-ID ingredients (NID) = 5 count

*All NID ingredients shorten digestion cycles and interrupt nutrition extraction. A meal may include several NID ingredients. Each individual NID = 5 count.

Example: Glass of conventional wine + maple sugar + another processed sugar (in a dessert) = 5+5+5 = Total 15.

Note: This is half the daily ingredient quota on the ID1 program.

Salt *(AVOID)

= 5 count/per incident* [After 1 teaspoon/day allowed]
*Salt is both a mineral ingredient and a preserving agent. *Note:* This is a NID food because overconsumption can elevate blood pressure and increase joint inflammation. Salt and salt substitutes are highly refined, delivering a more severe biological impact. Pink Himalayan salt* is acceptable, but only if it is under-processed. All salt consumption (unrefined and refined) should be limited to one teaspoon per day, or should otherwise be avoided.

*Note: Sea and table salts are heavily processed to remove residues. (AVOID)

Generational Grains/Flours*(AVOID)

= 5 count/per new grain or flour incident*

Generational grains are highly processed and commercially manipulated at the seedling phase. They also take longer to digest because most varieties have been created or grown using pesticides and fertilizers. Most grains would be affected, including organic and gluten free. See page 195 for more about generational grains.

୫୦ ୯୪

Heat treated oils* (AVOID)

= 5 count per incident*

Counting example: Vegetable oil + hydrogenated fat = 5+5= Total 10

୫୦ ୯୪

Sugars* (AVOID)

= 5 count per incident*

*All forms.

Processed sweeteners incite cravings, which increase the appetite.

Heat processed sugars (AVOID)

People eat too much sugar, and this is not always their fault. However, if the dieter is already overweight, extra sugar is not needed for energy, will not support weight-loss goals, and would most likely produce digestion anxiety. Because sugar is often an unavoidable ingredient, particularly when added to processed foods, consuming sugar automatically counts as a NID food.

The NID score for sugar is 5, which applies to each sugar type consumed during a single eating event, regardless of the variety. This NID is particularly severe because sugar is unsuspectingly found in random recipes. A more extensive section about sugar can be found on page 186.

ಬಂಞ

Alcohol* (AVOID)

   = 5 count per incident*

Alcohols produced today are made with processed ingredients. Commercially sold alcohols are made with added sulfurs, refined sugars, generational grains, and pesticide-sprayed fruit. All of these ingredients stimulate cravings and produce digestion anxiety. In addition, because of their high toxicity, commercial alcohols slow down overall digestion, quickly moving toxins to the liver, where they are converted to secondary fat. See page 227 for more about alcohols.

Off the chart NID's (AVOID) (NOT APPROVED)

*This category of "severe" toxins includes commercially made alcohols, chemically created medicines, and recreational drugs. When NID's are deliberately consumed, examples, smoking, alcoholism, and drug addiction, the threat to chronic illness rises because toxins gain immediate access to the bloodstream via the intestines and the liver. The key problem, highly processed toxins do not have complimentary enzymes, ensuring they will be under-digested and remain stored in the body as secondary fat.

Approved ingredients

Non-heated, under-processed fats*
= 2 count per incident

Examples: Virgin coconut oil, fresh lard (non commercial, wet-rendered), duck fat, avocados, ghee, olives, and unpasteurized nuts [pesticide-free preferred].

FREE(*) Ingredients

(*)Spices (under processed)

(*)Herbs (under processed)

(*)Fermented vegetables

(*)Coffee and teas (under-processed preferred)

(*)Espresso coffee (preferred)

(*)Green, herbal, and Kombucha teas (preferred)

(*)Organic coconut water

(*)Organic Kefir - limit to one cup per day

ಬಂ ಚಿ

Counting Examples

Example 2

Cheese sandwich = pasteurized dairy + generational grains (+salt) + butter. 5+5+(5)+5 =Total 20 (this total does not include additives).

Example 3

Thanksgiving dinner, including turkey and mash potatoes, and stuffing, and gravy, and green bean casserole, and cranberry sauce, and pumpkin pie, and rolls. The estimated total is 200+ ingredients, not including additives, preservatives and hormones. Note: This meal will take over 24 hours to completely digest, and will have a negligible nutritional impact. Most of the chemical additives would require special enzymes, which will not be immediately available, particularly when many ingredients are digested together.

৪০৫৪

Substitutions and Free(*) Ingredients

Sugar	Substitute: Organic Stevia.
Refined oils and fats	1. Substitute: Naturally occurring and unheated. 2. Oil sprays (for coating pans during cooking). These are highly processed. Use sparingly or avoid!
Salt	Substitute: Coconut aminos (*), Pink Himalayan salt. Use sparingly!
Non starchy vegetables	FREE (*) Preferred: Fresh, green, leafy. Cooked or raw.
Unripe fruit (edible)	FREE (*)
Herbs, spices, condiments	FREE (*) Except commercial ketchup, vinegars and mustards; these are highly acidic.
Liquid Aminos	FREE (*) Coconut preferred.

Illustration 4: Substitutes and Free Ingredients

Ingredients to eliminate or avoid

- On ID1—no grains or flour products for 120 days. Worth repeating. Most grains have been genetically modified as seeds, even those that are organic and gluten-free. The thorough digestion of grains is dependent on the overall quality of the seeds that make them. In addition, digesting grains can produce higher stomach acidity, which slows the overall rate of digestion.

- Avoid grain thickeners in gravies and sauces.

- Be aware of supplements made with starches and other fillers.

- For all plans, avoid heat-treated or pasteurized nuts (all types).

- Limit pasteurized ingredients (mostly dairy and nuts). Pasteurization is a form of flash heat treatment, which reduces a food's nutritional value, and destroys all naturally occurring enzymes.

- Although dairy has been given a lower ingredient count, avoiding this food for 120 days may improve overall digestion efficiency and expose allergy

156

symptoms. For probiotic support, one cup of organic plain yogurt or Kefir (a fermented dairy drink) is allowed.

୨୦ ୯୪

Allowed oils

Recommended oils include unrefined, raw, not heated, and organic oils. Spray oils contain synthetic and chemical additives, making them difficult to digest. Sprays are permitted, but these should be used only as they were designed, as a nonstick coating for cookware.

Any digestion anxiety caused after consuming synthetic and heat-treated fats will manifest as burping, gas, and severe stomachaches. To minimize these reactions, consume oils that are a natural part of the food, such as the fat found in non-pesticide avocados.

Most nuts are usually heat treated and/or pasteurized. However, nuts grown without chemical fertilizers, and not pasteurized, offer a digestion-friendly source of nutrition, fiber, and natural fat.

> **WHAT IS A RECIPE?**
> Recipes are ingredients or multiple foods combined to create a new food. This includes foods with added sugars, fat, and flavorings. In general, foods with combined ingredients will be poorly digested.

Tracking NID foods

NID ingredients are sometimes unavoidable, and more so if refined sugars and salt have been added to unsuspecting foods like yogurt, ketchup, and peanut butter. To avoid ingredient assumptions, read all food labels, especially when there are multiple, disguised, and combined varieties of sugar, salt, and fat.

If NID ingredients are being tracked in a weight-loss journal,** this type of tracking offers a personal record of ingredients, which do not support efficient digestion. This includes ingredients that may also initiate cravings and allergies.

Tracking NID foods also helps to identify those days and moments when binging is more frequent. Consuming indigestible NID foods can cause bouts of

158

digestion anxiety, and these reactions will become more obvious when they are being tracked.

> **Tracking allergies and cravings can improve weight loss. In the absence of a formal journal, tracking tools have been included in the Resources section.**
>
> ***A formal tracking and weight-loss journal is also available at valden.com.*

Ingredient reduction benefits include:

- Steady weight loss and fat removal, as well as reduced secondary fat accumulation over time.
- Increased digestion efficiency, particularly when there are fewer complex ingredients to digest.
- Fewer episodes of gas and physical discomfort when there is a reduction in overall digestion anxiety.
- Regular and smoother bowel movements—stool is firmer and less runny.
- A nutrition boost after adding more vitamin-rich foods.
- Improved pH management, which accelerates nutrient absorption, and strengthens the immunity.
- Increased consumption of not ripened fruit, adding more fiber, and limiting sugars in the overall diet.

- Reduction of heat-treated oils.
- Avoiding random sugars added to unsuspecting recipes.
- Cost-effective plan when there are fewer processed recipes and ingredients to buy.
- Better management of ingredients during social eating situations.
- Faster identification of hunger and craving triggers.
- Use of food tracking to identify destructive cravings and allergy-causing ingredients.

Social cravings

The following may be a familiar scenario. On a certain day, a certain irresistible food is eaten, for example, bagels, pizza, chips, or doughnuts. In an instant all that dedicated dieting focus (over weeks and months) is wiped away, and even worse, the dieter blames himself or herself for this craving lapse—which triggers more unnecessary eating. At this point the most important question is, what triggered these cravings?

It could be argued, the very act of dieting requires removing irresistible foods and replacing them with blander-tasting foods. However, eating "tasty" foods is a behavioral response promoted by society-specific eating routines. These could also be described as taste preferences, which have evolved over the course of a person's lifetime.

We respond to cravings because we choose to. If a person wants to eat a cookie, it is because he or she *wants* to eat a cookie, not because his or her body needs a cookie. If you learn only one thing from this book make it this, all cravings—sweet, sour, tasty, revolting, or culturally and socially influenced, are *emotional reactions* to food, not events the digestion understands.

In fact, the digestion couldn't care less about eating a cookie, because this food contains processed sugar, augmented fats, flour, and a host of preservatives, which the body is not equipped to thoroughly digest. In addition, these biologically inferior ingredients, particularly when they are combined together, have zero or nil nutritional value, and would not offer the level of nutrients needed to support long-term wellness.

When the foods we surrender to—cookies, bagels, potato chips, pretzels, pecan pie, cheesecake, and others, can be easily avoided, this is a signal that the taste buds are less stimulated. When this happens cravings are finally being recognized and managed.

80 CB

Review: Ingredient Management

The quantity of ingredients eaten should be sufficient to meet both nutritional and daily caloric needs. For example, eating ten apples during the open window is not healthy (or encouraged) because the body's nutritional needs cannot be met eating just one type of food. This also applies to high-protein diets, where eating excess protein could produce acid enzyme buildup, which over the course of time would cause bouts of indigestion, stomach pains—and

perhaps much worse.

Instead, eating a combination of highly

nutritious, simple-ingredient foods, can improve overall

digestion, as well as create a reliable digestion

infrastructure, which evenly and continuously

distributes high-quality nutrients.

ഇൻൽ

Organics – What's the point?

This depends largely on whether the organics are eaten exclusively, or combined with processed and engineered ingredients.

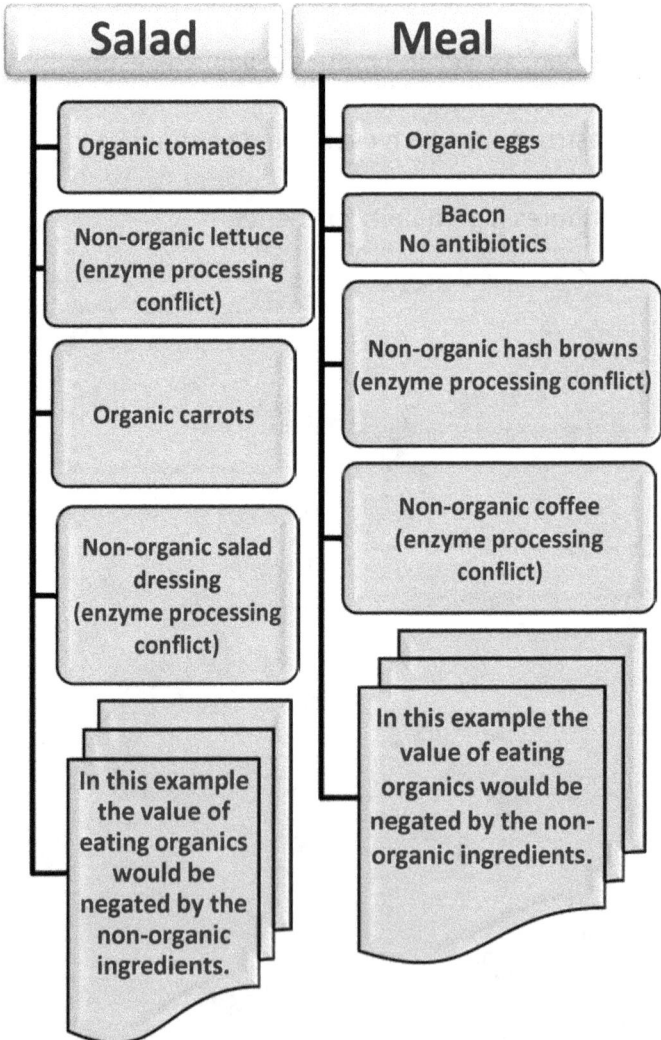

Salad

- Organic tomatoes
- Non-organic lettuce (enzyme processing conflict)
- Organic carrots
- Non-organic salad dressing (enzyme processing conflict)

In this example the value of eating organics would be negated by the non-organic ingredients.

Meal

- Organic eggs
- Bacon No antibiotics
- Non-organic hash browns (enzyme processing conflict)
- Non-organic coffee (enzyme processing conflict)

In this example the value of eating organics would be negated by the non-organic ingredients.

Chapter 8

The Digestion Drivers

Blood Factors

Genetics determines our blood type, resulting in blood chemistry varying from person to person. Other factors that alter blood chemistry include environmental impacts, culture, and water requirements. Serious health issues, including unexpected weight gain, may also be connected to deficiencies in overall blood composition or an abnormal pH. Improving blood pH can improve digestion efficiency, allowing the body more access to nutrients.

Not to be confused with blood type, which is also significant, the management of a healthy blood pH is usually dependent upon what a person eats, combined with overall digestion mechanics. These factors help to manage a person's overall health, where the blood's pH is viewed as the yin and yang of the circulatory system, allowing the balancing of elements, in this case either acid or alkaline, to dictate the overall health of the immunity.

Measuring pH

When foods are consumed and digested, the pH value is measured by an accumulating ash residue. This ash determines the overall pH impact of digested food on the blood. A negative pH, over acid or over alkaline, can be dangerous, particularly if this creates conditions, which allow unhealthy bacteria to thrive.

Because the typical western diet consists mainly of acid-forming edibles (wheat, sugar, dairy, meat, heat-treated fats, and medicines), this ensures the blood chemistry is predominantly acidic. Specific to pH management, this would create a higher than normal acid-forming ash residue.

What further aggravates these conditions is consuming other acid-forming foods, including sodas and overly brewed teas and coffee. Another variable is the sheer variety of recipes made from acid-forming ingredients. This list of offenders includes the combining of many types of sugars and grains in different recipes.

Specific to commercial sugars (all types) eating these in excess can attract (and accumulate) unhealthy bacteria, which may later trigger diseases from simple Candida, to more chronic illnesses such as cancers. For those who are overweight and practice modern diets, some of these programs encourage eating acid-forming foods, including different sugars, heat treated oils, a wide variety of grains, and with more frequency, hormone-produced meat proteins. These foods cause the blood's chemistry to consistently remain in a higher acid range, impeding nutrient absorption.

Remember 74.1!

Measuring pH requires using a pH scale, which spans from zero to fourteen. Human blood stays in a narrow pH range, approximately 7.35 to 7.45. Excessively below or above this range stimulates symptoms of illness. If blood pH moves below 6.8 (excessively alkaline), or above 7.8 (excessively acid), human cells function less efficiently and will no longer be able to maintain natural immunity.

Chronic illnesses become activated in a blood environment that is out of pH balance. The introduction of pH-specific foods can keep the blood's pH within a healthier range by discouraging the accumulation of illness-causing bacteria. Unfortunately, pH numbers are never exact or precise because blood chemistry changes with every meal and the frequency of clock eating. In addition, any grouping of engineered ingredients and their accompanying additives would limit the body's ability to maintain a stable pH.

Tracking acidity

The body must maintain some level of acidity, which varies from person to person. However, when there is an overabundance of secondary fat across the body, it can be presumed both blood acidity and toxicity have reached unhealthy levels. By eating fewer acid-forming foods, and eliminating excess fat stores, the blood maintains a more stable pH range, which strengthens overall immunity. That said, it is important to pay attention to what and when foods are eaten. This requires paying closer attention to the pH of all foods, at the same time avoiding large accumulations of acid-rich foods.

Protein requirements

By human design a lean man has a body composition of roughly 15 percent bone, 45 percent muscle, and 15 percent fat. A lean woman (on average) has 12 percent bone, 35 percent muscle, and almost 30 percent fat.[7] As this relates to the skeleton, because muscle supports bone health, this suggests consuming sufficient (not excessive) amounts of easily digestible protein would be important to building and retaining muscle. Muscle is also an efficient mechanism for transporting nutrients to the bones and cells. Relative to digestion performance, building and keeping muscle helps maintain pH balance. Building lean and efficient muscle requires not only eating sufficient protein, but managing protein portions to ensure all proteins are thoroughly digested.

However, overuse of a high-protein diet could also lead to unhealthy pH conditions, where the exclusivity of eating large amounts of higher acidity protein draws the blood into a higher acid pH, interrupting the distribution of nutrients.

---

[7] Resource section: Advanced Human Nutrition

pH and aging

Proteins become more difficult to digest as we age. This happens because there is diminished hormone activity, which produces shortages of specific enzymes. The older the person the smaller the quantity of enzymes he or she produces. As this relates to long-term weight loss, a high-protein diet would always require complimentary enzymes. Without these available in sufficient supply, proteins would not be digested either efficiently or completely.

When pH shifts out of balance overall weight loss would be slower. In general, these diets are not suitable for everyone, particularly women entering menopause, where the aging process further diminishes hormone activity. Although weight loss might be achieved, increased acidity would cause toxicity levels to rise, producing a less robust immunity and the possibility of chronic illness in later years. Higher acidity can also destroy calcium, resulting in progressive bone loss.

Diet selection

The digestion relies on enzymes being available, and as a chief influencer, having these enzymes on hand can improve weight loss results. If a diet focuses exclusively on protein consumption (at least 60 percent or more) and fewer of the required enzymes are available, there would be more frequent incidents of partial digestion. This causes the blood's overall acidity to rise, and nutrients to be destroyed. When there are fewer enzymes this hinders nutrient absorption, which eventually debilitates the immunity. Enzyme shortages cause undigested foods to linger in the digestion tract, waiting for either fat storage to begin, or with more frequency, poorly digested foods to be converted to fat and waste.

pH imbalance

Too much protein in the diet can also result in enzyme overproduction, where stores of certain readily available enzymes, for example protease and peptidase,

172

flood the digestion. Because proteins are predominantly acidic, and these particular enzymes are acid supporting, the blood's balancing systems are forced to compensate by boosting alkaline. Keeping a slightly higher alkaline pH is important for maintaining a robust immunity against severe illness, as well as distributing nutrients without destroying them. However, when too many acid-correcting enzymes (mostly alkaline) infiltrate these systems, this type of imbalance destroys nutrients.

What about secondary fat?

When chemical additives (all acidic) are not efficiently digested, secondary fat (also acidic) becomes the ideal storage container for toxic debris. Because fat storage is an automated function, when secondary fat accumulates, toxin levels quickly rise, producing pH imbalance across the body.

However, it is important to remember that secondary fat is a body defender, and used specifically to protect the main organs (heart, lungs, and liver) against rising toxicity. Secondary fat is also used to transport toxins to remote areas of the body. Because this fat acts as a storage container, the remoteness of these containers makes them less accessible for immediate energy needs. This remoteness also guarantees accumulated secondary fat would be difficult to break down and remove, causing overall pH to become unstable.

pH complications

When pH complications arise, there may be unpleasant or painful reactions caused by blood over-acidity. For these reasons a rising pH (either acid or alkaline) could initiate a wide array of unexpected health issues. This includes unhealthy autoimmune responses, disease escalation, virus invasion, allergic reactions, and unexpected failures within different body systems.

Review: pH Pros and Cons

Pro: High-protein diets are typically more effective when the protein is consumed in smaller portions, allowing for completed digestion and greater nutrient extraction.

Pro: Related to pH balancing, preferred alkaline sources include green vegetables, under processed vegetable proteins (beans, legumes, seeds, pea protein, and others); and when needed to manage nutrient deficiencies, smaller portions of non-hormone derived meat, fish, and eggs.

Con: Because flesh proteins are deficient in fiber, eating them in excess can produce digestion slowdowns. These slowdowns result in secondary fat accumulation—and if these slowdowns become frequent, the probability of increased acid pH in the blood, followed by severe bouts of digestion anxiety.

Con: Poor digestion causes partially digested food to linger in the digestive track, potentially raising both acid pH and body toxicity.

Con: Eating too much flesh protein slows down digestion, potentially producing painful physical reactions, including stomachaches, constipation, and dehydration.

Con: Meat and dairy proteins require more water to complete digestion, particularly if they are eaten several times a day, and delivered to the digestion as part of multiple-ingredient recipes. Insufficient water (dehydration) could cause a concentration of acid in the blood, resulting in an undesirable higher acid pH.

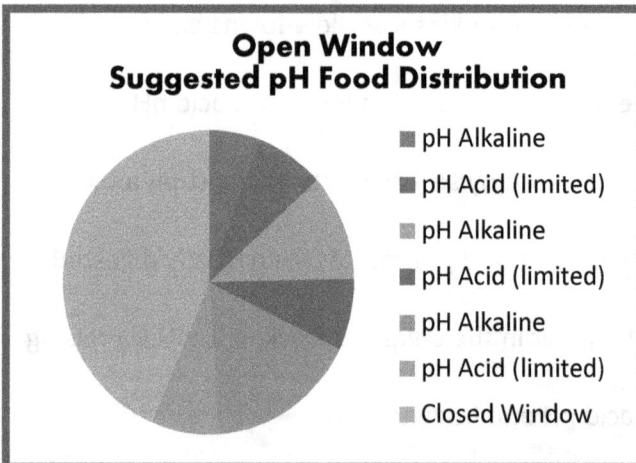

**Open Window
Suggested pH Food Distribution**

- pH Alkaline
- pH Acid (limited)
- pH Alkaline
- pH Acid (limited)
- pH Alkaline
- pH Acid (limited)
- Closed Window

Checking pH health[8]

*The following tool (see next page) can be used to evaluate pH imbalances. This is a purely subjective exercise, providing a personal snapshot of how eating certain foods could raise pH values. To assist with this assessment, pH food values have been included in the Resources section.

Complete this exercise at least twice a week to check overall pH.

Ø)CR

---

[8] Refer to pH charts in Resources section

The Ingredient Diet

What's my pH today?   Date:

1. Use the pH chart in the Resources section to add in the values). **Remember to first make copies!**

Breakfast		
Food 1	ACID	ALKALINE
Food 2	ACID	ALKALINE
Food 3	ACID	ALKALINE
Lunch		
Food 1	ACID	ALKALINE
Food 2	ACID	ALKALINE
Food 3	ACID	ALKALINE
Dinner		
Food 1	ACID	ALKALINE
Food 2	ACID	ALKALINE
Food 3	ACID	ALKALINE
Snack 1	ACID	ALKALINE
Snack 2	ACID	ALKALINE
Beverage 1	ACID	ALKALINE
Beverage 2	ACID	ALKALINE
Medications +Supplements	ACID	

2. **Circle** (below) any noticeable physical reactions after eating.
Burping; stomach pains; throat pain; allergies; acid reflux; out of sequence bowel movements; thirst.

Other: Add any reactions not listed above.

Note: All medications and supplements are assumed to be acidic.

Illustration 5: Daily pH Monitoring Tool/**Make copies!**

178

Chapter 9

The Best Ingredients?

> Which ingredients are the most genetically modified in the world's food supply?
> **The answer is...**
> **Almost all of them!**

Aggravators and accelerators

This chapter discusses individual ingredient categories, each afflicted by some form of food manipulation. The first ingredient classification is dairy.

Milk does it do a body good?

"Not only does pasteurization kill friendly bacteria, it also greatly diminishes the nutrient content of the milk. Pasteurized milk has up to a 66 percent loss of vitamins A, D and E. Vitamin C loss usually exceeds 50 percent. Heat affects water-soluble vitamins, and can make them 38 percent to 80 percent less effective. Vitamins B6 and B12 are completely destroyed during pasteurization. Pasteurization also destroys beneficial enzymes, antibodies and hormones. Pasteurization destroys lipase (an enzyme that breaks down fat), which impairs fat metabolism, and the ability to properly absorb fat-soluble vitamins A and D. (The dairy industry is aware of the diminished vitamin D content in commercial *milk*, so they fortify it with a form of this vitamin.)

We have all been led to believe that milk is a wonderful source of calcium, when in fact, pasteurization makes calcium and other minerals less available. Complete destruction of Phosphates is one method of testing to see if milk has been adequately pasteurized. Phosphates is essential for the absorption of calcium."

Resource: http://www.westonaprice.org

#1—Dairy

It seems ironic that raw milk is what humans have consumed for centuries without adverse effects. However, it is also true raw cow's milk carries potentially lethal bacteria.

Dairy products are not excluded from The Ingredient Diet. In fact, there is nothing wrong with consuming dairy—that is if the dairy is raw, unpasteurized, or comes from uncompromised milk. These conditions suggest digestible milk would have to come directly from cleanly managed, grass-fed cows, without sterilization, pasteurization, or added vitamin treatments.

So, why is milk pasteurized?

Death from foodborne illness is the greatest concern associated with consuming untreated dairy products. The accelerated rate of spoilage, and the time it takes to transport dairy across long distances, makes it necessary to pasteurize milk.

The U.S. government regulates milk production to safeguard people from illnesses. The full scope of government involvement requires managing all aspects of dairy farming including pasteurization methods and the different ways hormones are added to increase the milk supply. The government also regulates the additives used to bulk and fortify milk. This array of different treatments makes modern milk virtually incomparable to the milk consumed fifty or more years ago, and as a consequence, nutritionally deficient.

What happens during pasteurized?

Pasteurizing changes milk's molecular structure. These cellular alterations impact all milk products, including yogurt, cream, butter, and cheese. This process also reduces the lipase and calcium competency, while diminishing most of the naturally occurring probiotic enzymes. This is why pasteurized milk is often refortified with synthetic vitamins, to compensate for the natural vitamins lost during pasteurization.

Taking a break from dairy products, roughly 120 days, may not only reduce overall ingredients, but redirect the digestion so it breaks down more secondary fat. This

182

is a temporary reprieve, and implemented to observe

possible digestion problems. Don't worry, you can add

limited quantities of dairy back later—if you absolutely

have to!

Milk Substitutes
Popular milk substitutes are made with nuts or generational grains. Specific to nuts, these may be pasteurized, producing milks, which interact poorly with enzymes during digestion.

#2—Cravings

Ingredient monitoring and scaling back can help

reduce cravings. The body takes approximately 120 days

to recycle the blood (or 2, six week cycles on the ID1

plan). For the average dieter this time is better spent

giving up or significantly reducing oily, milky, sweet,

grain-rich, and salty foods. Based on the severity of

cravings, it may take longer than 120 days to experience

positive physical changes. The longer these ingredient

eliminations continue (multiple and consistent 6-week

cycles) the more noticeable health improvements will become.

#3—Allergies

There seems to be more allergens than ever before, and even more drugs created to subdue these symptoms. Making matters worse, medications created to relieve these symptoms are often chemically derived, and in most cases not permanent cures.

In general, allergies can be both curious and frightening. During the sixties allergic reactions to food were not as obvious as they are today, and the reasons for these adverse reactions, at least to the casual observer, are far from conclusive. The Ingredient Diet theorizes that food-specific allergic reactions happen when the body is unable to quickly digest the chemical agents used to create the foods eaten.

Offering one example, consuming peanuts, or even being near peanuts, may cause such a profound allergic reaction, where a person could actually die. To
184

clear up any confusion, peanuts are not nuts, they are seeds from a plant in the legume family, and legumes are just one of a subcategory of other foods, which include beans, lentils, alfalfa, clover, peas, carob, and soybeans. Most, if not all of these foods have been eaten by various cultures across the globe for centuries, and without adverse effects. In fact, many countries value peanuts because they are high in fiber and essential nutrients.

Similar allergic reactions have been observed after eating glutinous grains, engineered soy, and dairy products. Perhaps surprising, very severe allergy cases often occur in western cultures, where food-related complications arrive unexpectedly. Such coincidences may be connected to the ever-changing and different fertilizers and pesticides used to grow modified foods, which over the decades have changed the molecular structure of certain peanut crops, at least enough to produce unexpected and sometimes lethal digestion problems.

#4—Processed sugars

It seems somewhat ironic that the very substance that sustains humanity, blood glucose, is described by science as a form of sugar. Both humans and plants produce different forms of "sugar," but in the case of humans glucose is a convertible energy fuel, and as important as the very air they breathe.

However, when it comes to taste preferences, it is no secret that recipes with added sugar taste good, at least our cravings ensure this is the message our brains understand. Over the centuries our taste buds have been both enchanted and conditioned to eat more sugar, to the point where without sugar certain foods no longer taste palatable.

Food manufacturers have capitalized on our love affair by adding sugars (cane, honey, Stevia, and others) to recipes. These sugars are used not only to bulk up products, making them cheaper to produce, but more habitual, to appeal to our taste buds, thereby ensuring

186

repeat purchases. Making matters worse, sugar-packed foods such as sports drinks and supplement bars are promoted as auxiliary energy sources. Ironically, when given easily digestible, non-sugary foods, the human body can (in most situations) make its own energy fuel.

The body can also produce as much glucose as it needs. It can also sustain all basic physical functions for long periods of time using its fat reserves. Because of these unique biological mechanics, added sugars would not be needed for energy, except when there are medically diagnosed conditions related to blood sugar imbalances such as diabetes or hyperglycemia.

Specific to modern food manufacturing, many overly processed and multiple-ingredient recipes are made with a wide variety of different sugars. As this relates to digestion complexity, these modified sugars require more time to break down into simple components, and later be converted into glucose. When glucose is surplus, it is easily converted to fat, and most of this fat is viewed by the body as nonessential fuel. Other than a metabolic emergency, this fat would not be used for immediate energy needs, particularly when clock eating results in surplus glucose always being on hand.

What bees know

If the human body converts excess sugars into glucose, and then to fat, plants in contrast, convert their sugars to waste. Offering a contrarian perspective, when people consume plant sugars, this could be described as consuming a plant's by-products or waste.[9] Unlike glucose, which the body makes and uses for energy, many plant sugars, examples, cane, beet, and corn, do not manufacture sugar for the self-feeding of their creator plants. Instead, a small portion of these sugars are used by the plant for energy, while the greatest portion (the part people eat) would be eliminated as waste. This is a curious

---

[9] Recycling the Dead. Carbon activity in plant (dead) debris and waste. See Reference section.

188

aspect of plant biology, one that has been overlooked or ignored by most food manufacturers and modern science.

Sweeter fat

The body's fuel conversion and regulation process evaluates just how much non-glucose sugar can be absorbed, as well as how much of these sugars will be needed for energy. If the body already carries large reserves of fat, extra energy from extraneous sugars would be irrelevant to survival. Because this book is concerned with improving digestion performance, when a person is overweight, any oversaturation of glucose in the blood would be dealt with similar to toxic waste, removed and stored in remote areas of the body as stockpiles of natural fat.

Maintaining large reserves of circulating glucose also slows weight loss. That said, accelerating weight loss would require all surplus glucose to be exhausted. Because clock-eating is usually a frequent event, this guarantees glucose would always be surplus in the blood, resulting in slow and continuous fat gain over time.

To further complicate matters, when there are secondary fat stores across the entire body, most of these would not be easily accessible. These reserves could only be tapped during times of severe glucose depletion such as starvation, deliberate calorie reduction, or specific to The Ingredient Diet, during a closed window, when solid foods are not consumed for longer periods of time.

> *Don't be fooled! Processed sugars are hidden in something you ate today.*

Sweet eliminations

When improving digestion efficiency, refined and processed sugars are viewed as one of the leading health risk ingredients, and dangerous to the digestion if different sugars are added to complex recipes and commercially manufactured foods. That said, when using The Ingredient Diet the next critical elimination would be all varieties of added sugar, particularly those sugars that are overly refined.

Sugary pals

Most people are not aware of the large quantities of processed sugar they eat all day long. As a feature of lifestyle, sugars added to different recipes may be unavoidable. To better manage sweet cravings, isolating hidden sugars and monitoring food labels would be essential to avoiding both unexpected fat gain and toxin accumulation. Today processed sugars are added to cereals, breads, nutrition bars, packaged meats, cured meats, yogurt, peanut butter—and those are some of the healthier foods! When (and if) you give up sugar, this may require a deliberate and focused endeavor.

Moving away from a sugar-centered lifestyle would also require personally preparing the foods eaten, and gradually replacing sugar-added and "sugar-free" products with less sweet foods. When removing processed and refined sugars from the diet, this would involve making gradual adjustments. This includes scaling back on sweeter ingredients, while at the same time reducing portion sizes and eliminating the most obvious sugars first. Using a gradual reduction approach recalibrates the taste buds, allowing them to enjoy blander, less-sweetened foods.

Artificial sweeteners

There are many sweeteners on the market, and most of them are artificial. This description refers to sugars not derived from plant sources. Manufacturing artificial sugars involves combining chemicals and heat processing, which creates sweeteners with negligible nutrition prior to consumption. This category includes the sugar substitutes dextrose, sucrose, and aspartame. Eating these heat-treated foods produces immediate digestion anxiety.

Stevia—and whenever possible organic stevia, is an acceptable sweetener on the Ingredient Diet. Stevia is a plant leaf sweetener available from health food stores. As an approved ID ingredient, Stevia counts as a *free* food, whereas sugar has an NID of 5 per incident. However, consider limiting Stevia, as the sweet taste is considered a form of taste manipulation. Of course, unlike most artificial and chemically produced sweeteners, the taste of Stevia is not the same as sugarcane. Consider using Stevia as a tool to minimize sweet cravings.

Sugar research

Recent sugar-specific research, (see next section for video links) suggests that regularly consuming plant sugars is "safe or inconclusive." However, this research also indicates that when plant sugars are consumed in excess, this can result in an increase in blood lipoproteins, a major risk factor for cardiovascular disease.

If a plant eliminates its own sugars as a form of toxic waste, the human body responds similarly, rejecting plant sugars, and preferring glucose for its energy needs.

This also suggests consuming extraneous sugars may be toxic to the human body. As a self-preservation response, the digestion would immediately convert and store all surplus non sugars as secondary fat.

℘ℭℜ

The following research-based videos offer statistical data supporting the reasons why avoiding sugar could be beneficial to overall health. As a reminder, sugar consumption (all types), may play a key role in aggravating allergies, as well as contributing to heart disease and cancers.

A science-based perspective on how sugars negatively impact blood lipids.
1. High Sugar Diets and Disease; Dr. Kimber Stanhope, Department of Nutrition, UC Davis
https://www.youtube.com/watch?v=_AJka21yfyE

2. Fat, Fructose and FGF21—The Science Behind Fad Diets and Obesity; Patricia Chui, MD, Department of Surgery Grand Rounds, March 26, 2014
https://www.youtube.com/watch?v=YE4dlGrGPYk

Reference Section: 12 and 13

#5—Generational Grains

Bread has been part of the human diet since before the fifteenth century. Functionally, the idea of combining a few basic ingredients (grain flours, salt, and yeast) to make a filling and nutritious food is far from complex or outrageous. Eating a simply created food can also be comforting and filling.

Basic grains, associated grain ingredients, and grain recipes, are made with *generational grains* (all types—commercial, organic, and gluten free). This describes grain seeds, which during their lifespan have been manipulated by chemicals, fertilizers, and pesticides. Modern bread and bread-like products made with generational grains (examples, pancakes, cakes, tortillas, biscuits, and crepes) delay digestion. This is because the seeds that produced the original flours were already contaminated, and as a result, already nutritionally deficient.

Regular consumption of generational grain products would not only accelerate secondary fat

195

production and storage, but would most likely yield very little absorbable nutrition. All grains, including modern-day rice, corn, millet, wheat, and rye, are part of this category. The only exception would be grain products made from unadulterated grain seeds, which today would be difficult to find.

Grain products should be eaten sparingly. They have been added to this program to offer dietary variety, but modern grains are considered a cautionary ingredient.

#6—Cloning

As fewer poor quality ingredients are eaten, there will be a period of adjustment where cravings may be difficult to manage. Do your best! The objective is to remove chemically treated and overly processed ingredients from the overall diet. This may include certain foods you love or have grown up eating, particularly those carrying special memories.

Specific to these memories, the foods we enjoy may have a historic time stamp. However, along the way these were replaced by adaptations, which have manipulated our taste sensitivities. Being structurally and molecularly altered by modern manufacturing systems, these "clone" foods are inferior substitutes, not even close to the actual foods we once enjoyed.

ഇന്റ

#7—Water—The best ingredient!

Drinking water could be described as the most important digestion aligning tool. In the typical western diet, where most foods are less moist, mostly acid pH, and eaten frequently (as a feature of clock eating) these variables require drinking even more water, at least enough to move poorly digested foods through the various digestion cycles.

The amount of water a person drinks is unique to each individual. This amount varies depending on factors such as gender, what his or her activity level is, and what climate zone he or she lives in. Beyond managing thirst, maintaining correct water levels allows the body to better manage biological functioning. Drinking water also improves nutrition delivery systems by flushing out toxins, which is a feature of efficient blood circulation.

How much water to drink?

Based on those factors already described, the average daily water requirement also depends on the amount of physical energy exerted. To compensate for perspiration loss, and especially for those who are overly active, or exercise regularly, this would call for consuming more water than the minimum. That said, there would always be a daily required amount needed to manage overall digestion mechanics.

Unnaturally lower levels of water in the body, or becoming dehydrated, would cause the metabolism to slowdown, further interrupting the speed of fat loss and weight loss. Finally, the inability to identify thirst could

198

ignite cravings for sugary and salty foods, while drinking the correct amounts of water would discourage cravings.

Water quotas do not include the water found in other beverages, particularly when added ingredients would require more comprehensive digestion. To ensure the thorough digestion of all foods, an ingredient-rich diet, chock-full of sugar, salt, fillers, preservatives, and hormones, would require more water than the usual quotas.

⧖⧗

Rule of Thumb: Even when not dieting, drink daily 10/8-ounce glasses of pure water.
(This would be the absolute minimum)

Drinking water – The golden rules

- For most adults the recommended rule is to drink eighty ounces of water a day, or 10/8-ounce glasses. More water would be needed if a person was overly active, or performed vigorous exercise, or ate an ingredient-rich diet.

- The best way to drink water is to "sip and chew," which engages the digestion and activates enzymes in the mouth and stomach. Take a sip; then slush or chew the water for a few seconds; then swallow.

- Alternately, drinking too much water during meals dilutes enzymes, resulting in poor digestion outcomes.

- Drinking pure water, without other foods and beverages, avoids the full digestion process, while offering a more efficient form of rehydration.

- There is no substitute for drinking pure, clean water. Beverages, juices, or consuming large quantities of fruit and vegetables, would not count as part of the daily water quota. This is because these foods have to undergo complete digestion.

- A physical water shortage (dehydration) delays the response to feeling full, which activates premature hunger and cravings.

- Drinking enough water helps to rid the body of fat and toxins, improving weight loss results over time.

Part II

Minding the Future

Part II addresses chronic health issues associated with digestion inefficiencies. Perhaps surprising, this includes both a decline in human learning, and an increase in incidents of mental illness across all adult age bands.

Whether intentional or not, the dumbing down of humanity may be related to modern food regulatory practices, as well as new recipe innovations.

Chapter 10

Digestion and Critical Thinking

> **Did you know eating too many processed foods could cause the mind to become less focused on managing overall health?**

If nutrition absorption becomes impaired, and the digestive system does not operate at peak, the brain cannot be relied upon to manage the body's nerves and other sensors. These unhealthy biological circumstances also interrupt decision-making, which not only influences daily cognition, but may extend to other social problems, including criminal behaviors, diminished scholastic aptitude, drug abuse, and the rapid decline of mental health—all of these impacting different adult and juvenile age bands.

If the nutrition delivery system becomes impaired, both the physical and mental sensory mechanisms decline together. When this decline continues across consecutive decades, it would become difficult for the digestion and other body systems to efficiently manage overall health. Because the taste buds are a small part of a larger sensory mechanism, when taste sensitivities are exposed to nutritionally deficient ingredients for long periods of time, the appetite for poor quality food increases. This happens because eating meals activates ingredient-sensitive cravings—perhaps many times during a day. This is one example of the mind and body communicating poorly, and these are the same communications managing overall health.

Learning problems

Granted, a poor education system might be to blame for certain students not doing well in various school systems. However, could eating poor quality food also be a disabling factor? The latest and most stirring cognition-related concern is the decline in learning functions affecting young people. The data collected examined advanced nations such as the United States, and tracked academic test performance across recent decades.[10] This data also compared the test scores of similar students in other countries. The United States showed a noticeable decline in academic performance affecting numerous age bands, but the greatest impact was observed in teens and young adult students. Of further concern, this decline was not isolated to core subjects like math and English, but a wide variety of subjects.

Although nationally compiled data showed small academic gains for grades four to eight, older American

---

[10] Data available in Reference section Page 251.

students did not fare as well when compared to their international counterparts. Again, this declining trend was more prevalent in older students, and may have something to do with the time it takes for nutrient deficiencies to impact cognition performance, combined with the quantity of processed foods these students have eaten during their lifetime.

Here the unanswered question is, could genetic and cognitive decline be connected to poor digestion performance? This would be the gradual degeneration of cognition competency, which includes reduced literacy and learning aptitude caused by nutrition deficiencies.

ಶೂ ಛಾ

Mental Health Equation
●   ●   ●
Over stimulated taste buds = Decreased cognition over time.

The smarter ones

Another concern is the decline in intelligence, concentration, focus, and the inability to learn functional skills. These issues appear more prevalent in parts of the world where eating processed foods would be culturally ingrained across generations, and societies are conditioned to recognize processed foods as being a reliable source of nutrition. Coincidentally, these happen to be pockets of the world where there is also a prevalence of obesity, diabetes, and cancer.

If these social and health-related issues are linked to consuming refined and engineered foods, relying on academic data alone would be insufficient to identify the full spectrum of disabling cognition-related factors impacting many different age bands.

૪ ૭

Cognition and aging

In North America, dementia has been diagnosed in adults in their thirties.[11] This form of early cognitive degeneration may be connected to eating larger quantities of nutritionally-deficient foods before reaching high school age, and this trend continuing through maturity. Because engineered foods have been in circulation since the 1950's, cognitive degeneration could be symptomatic of a genetic decline affecting multiple generations.

Witnessing the genetic consequences

Similar concerns may be linked to rising birth defects, increased premature births, and most obvious, evidence of infertility in young, healthy adults. It is also not uncommon to find couples seeking infertility treatments, or exploring adoption programs, after multiple, complicated, and difficult pregnancies. It would

---

[11] Dementia Now Afflicting People in Their 40s as Mercury from Vaccines Causes Slow, Degenerative Brain Damage

appear poor digestion issues may have far-reaching biological consequences.

Not surprising, the response from the scientific community has been to monetize these problems. This has sparked the growth of a birth and fertilization industry focused on artificial baby-making innovations such as sperm banks and in-vitro fertilization. These methods use chemically-created drugs to stimulate male and female hormones. These are drugs specifically designed to resuscitate what is often diagnosed by doctors as stagnant reproduction.

Disease prevalence

Beyond mental disease and reproduction issues, is the curious escalation of incidents of chronic illness. Cancers have become relatively common health issues, and they seem to be increasing by both type and frequency. This particular category of diseases rapidly deteriorates the immune system, making it difficult to isolate the root cause and discover permanent cures.

Cancers also appear to be more prevalent in societies consuming larger quantities of processed and ingredient-rich food. Because processed foods have changed over time (using newer and stronger chemical additives, fertilizers, and hormones) the isolation and cure of these severe illnesses has become elusive. Interesting to note, when it comes to combating mutating diseases, surgical innovations have shown to be more successful when compared to the overuse of unstable pharmaceutical drug cocktails.

Where science-based strategies seem to be unpredictable, perhaps the only reliable intervention would be a departure from chemical treatments, instead finding alternative ways to nourish the cells of the organic body. Ideally, this would involve replacing "curing" drugs with nutrient dense foods, thereby fortifying the immunity so it could heal and repair itself. Unfortunately, this would also rely on a revision of food quality standards, including modifications to many chemically-created ingredients. If

210

these standards are not addressed soon, incidents of

unexpected sickness will continue to escalate.

> **Providing a general definition, a full-fledged cure would be a remedy that could cure everyone who contracted the same disease or illness in the same or identical way.**

Curing disease

Regardless of costly medical breakthroughs, which

seem more temporary than permanent, there have been

few absolute cures for any serious health disorders in the

last fifty years. Furthermore, once diagnosed, many

people die rather than survive, and this is often preceded

by a painful and prolonged period of illness. These health

circumstances affect the young and the old, and all

cultural groups.

It would appear that even with medical and

scientific advancements, very few will survive chronic

illness. In contrast, any survivors of severe illness could be

considered unique cases, particularly when they are not

recipients of a global cure. As we eat more and more

modified and engineered foods, incurable diseases will most likely become more severe and untreatable—which is already happening.

ॐ

The following chart represents disease escalation over time. Most of these diseases have no permanent remedy.

CAUSES OF DEATH (WORLDWIDE) - Estimates for 2000-2012				
	2000		ESCALATION 2012	
	Females Age 0-70+	Males Age 0-70+	Females Age 0-70+	Males Age 0-70+
	All ages (total) years	All ages (total) years	All ages (total) years	All ages (total) years
Nutritional deficiencies	12477	6822	14224	8405
Iron-deficiency anemia	4932	2508	6361	3682
Malignant neoplasm	1186152	1472986	1318775	1648362
Cancer - Mouth and or pharynx	13865	47506	16733	53129
Cancer - Esophagus	15953	52898	16902	61308
Cancer - Stomach	85540	128656	72157	115396
Cancer - Colon and rectum	163194	167970	171565	192894
Cancer - Liver	36816	68893	43849	82118
Cancer - Pancreas	68343	69636	93179	95522
Cancer - Trachea, bronchus, lung	164495	412118	214527	432780

Cancer - Melanoma and other skin	17997	22588	**22730**	**32721**
Cancer - Breast	204401	0	**215641**	0
Cancer - Cervix uteri	37847	0	37483	0
Cancer - Ovary	61920	0	**66646**	0
Cancer - Prostate	0	136471	0	**157658**
Cancer - Bladder	20437	53444	**23268**	**65316**
Alzheimer's disease and other dementias	143126?	63163?	**366553?**	**173778?**
Cardiovascular diseases	3063299	2517528	2793778	2381857
Hypertensive heart disease	117644	71029	**176547**	**113257**
Stroke	1008299	652287	831094	574354
Cardiomyopathy, myocarditis, endocarditis	59567	84678	**62675**	**87560**
Respiratory diseases	248387	339335	**289366**	**360332**
Digestive diseases	212867	255059	**249854**	**297039**
Peptic ulcer disease	18310	23721	14961	20074
Cirrhosis of the liver	62998	121410	**76974**	**137020**
Kidney diseases	67663	63099	**92832**	**85916**
Down's syndrome	1481	1398	**1833?**	**1935?**

*Illustration 6:(Repeated from page 18) World Health Organization (WHO) 2015 /See Resources for website. ***Bold** *represents an increase in disease prevalence over time. 100K increments.*

Prescription ingredients

A rising disease backdrop suggests that the human biology (considered by many as the most superior organism on this planet) is now unable to find self-repairing solutions for many modern health issues. Based on the Ingredient Diet premise, global health will continue to debilitate, particularly if the body is unable to recognize how to adequately digest food and extract enough nutrition to nourish itself.

Based on these circumstances, medical interventions requiring specific drug interactions would only be effective for short periods of time. This may be why prescription drugs are constantly changing, with doses being adjusted higher rather than lower. If the digestion is forced to break down complex medications, hormones, and preservatives, in most situations the full spectrum of enzymes needed would not be available during the typical digestion cycle.

Because of these ever-changing biological conditions, most drug interventions (not surgeries) become interim solutions and not permanent cures. This also suggests the length of time a drug is reliable depends on the availability and quantity of digestive enzymes, and how these enzymes interact with chemically-created medicines, as they digest with chemically-created foods.

The guardians of food?

The greatest threat to human evolution appears to be the impact of poor quality nutrition on diminishing intellect. That said, the mind's ability to make better food choices becomes critical to safeguarding intelligence, mental health, overall wellness, and illness recovery. Delving deeper requires examining a wide range of food-related obstacles. The first is the sheer quantity of processed foods on offer. This includes engineered ingredient combinations, as well as the manipulation of a wide range of food recipes.

Of equal concern, engineered ingredients are approved after they have met mediocre government guidelines, ensuring they reach consumers (and food manufacturers) in record time. This suggests government regulatory organizations are ill-equipped to properly investigate the biological certainty of ingredient combinations, particularly when certain chemically-created ingredients combine with other chemically-created ingredients during digestion. This irresponsible and harmful regulation posture persists even as chronic illness and escalating ill-health continue to rise, and with only second-rate (mostly chemical) remedies on offer.

Specific to the present-day escalation of disease, the food safeguards worldwide governments have put into place appear to be biologically inadequate. Specific to the United States, and the revision of the Food Pyramid in 2011, this government-created dietary tool does not include processed and engineered ingredients, even when these foods are consumed by large sectors of the overall

216

population. This suggests the existing Food Pyramid, whichever way it is inverted, is an unreliable (and inaccurate) health-monitoring tool.

Regulations

For decades we have been told by various world governments, researchers, and food industry experts, that manufactured and refined foods are safe to eat, even "good for us," but this may not be the whole truth; at least not based on the level of refinement and the combining of ingredients, which has increased from decade to decade.

Even as we revisit diets tried and failed, perhaps some of these programs might have been effective if the recommended foods and ingredients had not been modified, and as a consequence, been incompatible with digestion processing.

Review: The dots align

Not all modern health issues appear to come from diseases passed down by our ancestors. In fact, our forefathers may have been genetically healthier, with a greater aptitude for learning than the generations that have followed.

The overly managed foods people eat may contribute not only to severe illnesses, but also to premature aging, infertility, cognition problems, autoimmune diseases, genetic abnormalities, and the decline of intellectual aptitude. Intellectual aptitude also appears to show a sharper decline in low, socioeconomic and urban neighborhoods, where geographically isolated students struggle academically. Coincidentally, these are the same neighborhoods where there is a prevalence of poverty and illiteracy, and where the vast majority of foods and recipes eaten are overly processed, overly manufactured, and derived from high ingredient counts.

∽∞∝

Chapter 11

At Our Expense

Many of today's weight gain and chronic illness

problems include food allergies, some so unique that

they cannot be properly identified using allergy testing.

Because people are genetically different, how they

digest food (and certain ingredients) may also be

uniquely different. These interactions may be the

reason why many allergies cannot be easily identified.

Weight loss interruptions

If adverse allergies are food counter reactions, for

those trying to lose weight, dieting may have become a

frustrating and lifelong preoccupation. If poor digestion

conditions persist, certain unfit ingredients would first

have to be removed from the overall diet to achieve

weight loss and wellness goals. This requires a change in

eating behaviors, or more specifically, a change in eating

routines to minimize poor ingredient interactions.

However, when taking a cursory look at the entire

food supply system, there is no mistaking that most, if not

all consumed ingredients, are in some way modified or

engineered. These are food systems where each part is

connected to another, compromising the quality of all

foods and ingredients within each system. This is a hard

fact to acknowledge, particularly when most of us believe

the foods we eat are safe, and safeguarded by various

trusted authorities.

Major challenges ahead

Attempting to change the processed food industry

would be a monumental undertaking, one that our

governments and other food regulating agencies are not

financially or administratively prepared to take on. In

addition, it is not possible to reconstruct the entire

220

commercial food system, particularly when there are so many processed, engineered, and overly refined ingredients in circulation.

Because food manufacturers are often focused on turning profits, they cannot be relied upon to make the necessary improvements to ensure biological food safety. Considering the wide variety of foods produced with additives, preservatives, pesticides, fillers, and hormones, these foods would first have to be reengineered to conform to new regulatory guidelines. If this happened—probably not in our lifetime, the cost of food would spiral out of control, causing financial hardship, especially for those low-income consumers who rely on access to affordable foods to make ends meet.

Healthy foods—the expensive myth

A dramatic increase in incidents of chronic disease, and the corresponding global awareness linked to this, has prompted the popularity of health food markets, which today are viewed as a reliable alternative to commercial food vendors. This began as a legitimate effort to elevate health consciousness, at the same time offering the public more access to higher quality nutrition. However, in recent decades even health foods are manufactured using a wide array of regulatory guidelines. It would appear that our understanding of natural and healthy has become manipulated by commercialism and governing rules. Beyond manufacturing regulations, at least these markets offer consumers access to larger varieties of naturally derived ingredients.

ॐ 03

Ingredient imposters

One unanticipated response has come from the commercial food industry. Not wanting to miss out on a windfall of profits, and fully aware of a shift in consumer loyalty, this industry has introduced "healthier" versions of already existing, refined, and processed foods. This includes everyday staple foods like low fat yogurts, and "all natural" cereals. This is yet another form of food manipulation, where ingredient integrity suffers, and the human digestion is exposed to a wider variety of nutrient deficient foods.

> **If a small segment of the world's population has access to "all natural" foods, what is everybody else eating?**

Broken receptors

With so much indigestible nutrition in the world's food supply, the first biological impact would be sensory damage, which might easily be overlooked, particularly if symptoms of ill health are not obvious. For example, eating a fresh apple, and deciding if the taste of this food was not mouth-watering or tasty would be a poor sensory decision. This is why many of us who live in advanced western cultures prefer to eat candy, cheesecake, and cookies, versus fresh fruit for dessert. In this example the nutritional quality of both options is incomparable.

In contrast, more reliable taste bud objectivity is observed from strict vegetarians and vegans, whose food choices gravitate toward blander tasting salads and undercooked vegetation. These individuals experience fewer cravings, and might actually get excited and salivate when they describe eating vegetables. In contrast, based on growing demand, people living in highly populated areas experience cravings for sugary, salty, baked, and fried foods.

The way forward

In recent times greater food quality awareness has blossomed, particularly when linked to the threat of illness. Unfortunately, healthier food options are not always available to the vast majority, including communities living in impoverished conditions. Even in the United States, where food is plentiful, not all consumers have access to affordable, high quality nutrition.

Based on those conditions already described, poor digestion appears to be a circumstance not solely connected with issues of wealth or poverty, but primarily food manipulation. As we continue to sacrifice nutrition for taste, we are left to witness either personally or globally, a rise in obesity, hypertension, diabetes, and many new incurable diseases. Further unfortunate, the ongoing dilemma between profits and health will continue to stymie research advancements, particularly when it comes to finding consistently reliable, non-chemical cures.

ଊ ଓ

Sensory taste alignment happens when:

1. The body gains continuous access to high quality and easily digestible nutrition.

2. The individual installs nutrition-focused eating behaviors.

3. Taste objectivity is recovered, followed by efficient digestion, minimized cravings, improved weight loss, and consistent lifelong wellness.

Chapter 12

The Enforcers

ॐ⃝

The final section of this book presents a series of independent observations describing uncommon digestion issues.

ॐ⃝

Alcohol—shaken, not stirred!

Alcohol was invented many centuries ago.

Believe it or not, this beverage was created to provide

wellness benefits. The water supply in olden times was

not as sanitary or abundant as it is today, and

fermented drinks became a popular alternative

because they did not spoil, and could be easily

transported. These alcohols include medicinal wines

and brandies, made in small batches, and from naturally derived ingredients.

In contrast, many modern-day alcohols are manufactured using refined and engineered grains and sugars. Even prior to processing the beneficial fermentation advantages are reduced, leaving the final consumer product stripped of vital nutrients. These refinements also increase the alcohol content and unleash a lethal killer—surplus sugar alcohol.

Having higher levels of sugar alcohol, as well as being both chemically engineered and mass-produced, ensures these alcohols also have a higher acid pH. This allows them to easily bypass the full digestion process, moving directly to the liver, the organ viewed by the digestion as the natural defender of body toxicity. Coincidentally, the liver is also the organ responsible for managing the distribution of both natural fat and secondary fat. When there are larger fat reserves on hand, new fat is quickly sorted, removed, and stored about the lower extremities of the body (lower abdomen, thighs, hips and buttocks). However, in recent decades an overabundance of toxins in the bloodstream has forced the various biological systems to transport secondary fat across the entire body.

More about salt

As previously mentioned, salt was one of the world's first preservatives. Today, salt is liberally used in processed foods as a preserving agent. Similar to processed sugar, salt can be labeled (or disguised) in many different ways. However, unlike sugar, salt contains minerals, giving it a modicum of nutritional value. The danger lies in how much the salt has been refined, and for some individuals the overconsumption of refined salt could trigger high blood pressure and water retention. Alternatively, too little salt could contribute to dehydration. Considering these variables, limiting salt as an ingredient becomes a double-edged sword. If unsure what salt quantities are safe, a medical doctor can provide more reliable usage guidelines, particularly if serious health-related problems exist.

Fruit controversy

Accessing the nutrition in fruit depends on whether the nutrients in the fruit can be absorbed by the body. Historically, fruits are grown given the climate and the season. This is significant to the digestion because the enzymes available to digest fruit depend on differing conditions, including climate changes, a person's genetic history, where they were born, and where their ancestors were born. For those hailing from tropical climates, these individuals may have more of the required enzymes needed to access the nutrients in fruit grown in these regions. Based on these assumptions, Europeans and North Americans would be less likely to have similar stomach enzymes or strength in enzymes, causing the nutrients in tropical fruits to be less accessible.

Specific to commercial fruit manufacturing, in recent decades certain fruits are grown all year round using synthetic growing agents. By eating fruit out of season, not to mention fruits already manipulated by fertilizers and pesticides, these circumstances may not result in complete or thorough digestion, and further reduce nutrition distribution.

ℬℭ

Because addiction is a larger topic than the scope of this book, it has been included next to offer possible reasons why addicts are unable to stop ingredient-specific addictive behaviors. In most situations, if not too late for intervention, using a dietary strategy, which adds more high quality nutrition to the overall diet, may encourage faster recovery.

Why are addictions on the rise?

Many addictions involve edibles, which must be digested. With no research pointing to a mutual cause, smoking, alcoholism, drug-related abuses, and certain mental disorders, could be connected to nutrient deficiencies. These addictions may occur because the digestion and sensory mechanisms become impaired at the same time, causing abrupt taste distortions, which lead to further drug abuse. In recent decades the rate of addiction has increased, and may be indirectly linked to advancements in food manufacturing, coupled with the quantity of poor quality ingredients the addict consumes over their lifetime.

When someone becomes addicted, their sensory taste mechanism has already become disabled, and is unable to signal the brain to stop these behaviors. As a consequence, eating nutrient-dense or high-quality food is no longer important to the addict, and any prolonged abuse of stimulants causes the addict's body to become further vulnerable to their addiction.

Finally, almost all addiction stimulants are heavily processed, and the stimulants of choice (drugs, nicotine, prescription medications, refined sugars, alcohols, and more) are engineered to such a degree, they may be viewed by the body as indigestible. Also, because most stimulants cannot be properly matched with complimentary digestive enzymes (they just don't exist) they bypass the full digestion process, moving to the liver to be stored as secondary fat. This is the worst possible scenario for the addict, particularly when the liver offers a direct gateway into the blood stream.

Beyond the threat of neurological and emotional damage, as body toxicity rises, the sensory mechanism becomes further disabled, and to such a degree where recovery would take longer, be difficult to manage, and based on the progression of the addiction, may never happen. These circumstances suggest modern treatments such as medications and psychological interventions would not be reliable, solo, long term solutions. This may be why the rate of addiction continues to climb.

Aging

Perhaps not obvious until too late, the nutrient delivery systems have a relationship to how we are visually acknowledged. Boosting digestible nutrition can help repair cell damage, slow the graying of the hair, strengthen the bones and joints, and increase the luminosity and moisture of the complexion. If the body is not receiving enough nutrition, it is likely aging will be premature. Not only will people age internally, they will also appear older sooner.

Our beloved pets

In recent decades the pet food industry has over-marketed the nutrition offered in dry, overly processed, and refined pet foods. Many dried food brands are made with generational grains, including, soy, oats, corn, rice, and wheat, to name just a few. Coincidentally, all of these ingredients are not only dry, but highly refined.

More and more of our beloved pets are eating indigestible ingredients, and as a consequence, nutrient-deficient foods. Most surprising, these dry foods are promoted by trusted veterinarians as being the finest source of nutrients. What often goes unnoticed, each year more domestic animals are being diagnosed with weight gain, urinary infections, leukemia, tumors, cancers, kidney failure, and blood disorders. Also not obvious, animals eating a dried food diet would experience the same digestion deficiencies as humans, where indigestible ingredients become converted to toxic secondary fat, and later stored somewhere in the body.

Another pet-specific digestion issue, dry foods must be rehydrated so they can be thoroughly digested, and this requires the animal to drink more water than they probably do. If this does not happen, the pet becomes dehydrated, which may lead to future kidney and urinary problems.

The last major issue would be the same for humans, the animal's digestion system has to find the correct sequence of enzymes to break down the preservatives and hormones within overly processed and engineered ingredients. Over time, poor digestion and nutrient absorption result in unavoidable health issues. These will not be easy to cure, costly to manage, shorten the life span of the pet, and as an unforeseen consequence, produce unexpected suffering.

෪෬

Suggestion: To keep pets healthier, feed them a nutritionally sound diet filled with nutrient dense, digestible, moist, and under-processed ingredients.

Celebrations—the best till last!

Of course, we must celebrate when opportunities present themselves. The question is how to celebrate with engineered food and stay healthy? Unfortunately, many modern food celebrations include highly processed recipes made with multiple ingredients, generational grains, hormone-derived meats, pasteurized dairy, processed sugars, heat-treated oils, overly refined salt, and chemically derived preserving agents.

Paying attention and planning for upcoming food-centered events would require predicting menus and avoiding recipes, particularly when certain unfit ingredients are not obvious or cannot be counted accurately.

Celebration tips

1. Ahead of the food event, anticipate the options and plan accordingly.

2. At the event, take the time to make the best nutrition choices.

3. When attending brunches and buffets, eat before arriving.

4. At the event begin by piling your plate with fresh vegetables, and then adding limited amounts of uncompromised protein.

5. These are events where generational grain recipes would be avoided to improve overall digestion efficiency.

಼ഐ ഒ಼

TIP: When visiting restaurants, the final menu choices are not determined by the menu selections, but by the highest nutrition choices available.

The balancing act

The benefits and pitfalls of dieting appear infinite. For example, in the early stages of The Ingredient Diet a cause of genuine anxiety might be giving up routine meals. In contrast, the benefits of a nutrition-focused diet (not immediately obvious) would include the gradual easing of bloating and gas, fewer allergic responses after minimizing gluten and pasteurized dairy, and longer sleep cycles, contributing to more physical rest. These are just a few of the positive physical responses experienced after the body receives more digestible nutrition.

Using the ID1 and ID2 plans can install an independence from clock eating, limit poor quality ingredients, and manage cravings. However, with any sensible eating plan, the objective would be to change both mental and physical responses to how food is consumed, particularly when absorbable nutrition has been absent from the diet for years and decades.

Finally, most diets fail because dieters forget their objectives and diet goals. Rereading Chapters 6 and 7 every thirty days can help maintain diet momentum and ensure more consistent weight loss over time.

ಬಿ ಲ

Maintain diet goals by:

- Writing down and continually adjusting goals.
- Posting goals with target dates on a calendar or to-do list.
- Updating goals when targets are reached (or not).
- Using a fat loss scale for tracking fat lost.
- Using pH strips to monitor over-acidity in the blood.
- Recording improved health markers, including, less gas and bloating, better sleep cycles, reduced joint pain, increased energy, and consistent weight lost.
- Tracking and monitoring results in a weight loss journal, ** even if they are initially slower than expected.

**A weight loss tracking journal is available at valden.com.

Review: Basic ID diet pointers

- Move away from recipes with over 8-10 ingredients.
- Avoid ingredients made with refined sugars and salt.

- Avoid foods that require the body to rehydrate them prior to digestion, this includes pasteurized nuts and large portions of meat.
- Manage over-acidity by eating a higher percentage of alkaline foods.

ℛℭ

The hopeful finale!

This ingredient management program introduces a wellness strategy, which attempts to maneuver a very complicated and unfortunate series of food-related circumstances. Eliminating scheduled meals, complex recipes, and improving digestion efficiency, become the top priorities. The next phase involves removing heat-treated oils, sugars, high-acidity foods, and overly processed ingredients. These ingredients will either be out of your life for good, or scaled back to such a degree where the effect on the digestive system is minimal.

Greater lifelong physical awareness and having a stronger immunity will be the natural outcomes of completed digestion cycles. Far more important, the best nutrition choices will foster heightened intelligence, mind clarity, and support a body that knows how to efficiently energize and heal itself.

Eat nutritious foods.

Manage ingredient quality.

Lose fat.

Stay well.

Live longer!

The longer we eat processed, refined, and combined ingredients, the more our health and intelligence as a population of people on this planet will decline.

Appendix

Not a myth - there is proof

Cognition and Declining Test Scores

"Student scores on standardized tests have steadily declined since 1965. Researchers conducted a literature review and completed data analysis to determine the reasons for this decrease, assessing trends for the period from 1965 to 1983. The kinds of tests most commonly used are aptitude, achievement, and tests of personal and social characteristics. Score trends vary from test to test. The reasons for the declining student scores include changes in the composition of test-takers, decreases in the quantity of schooling which students experience, curriculum changes, declines in student motivation, and deterioration of the family system and social environment. These factors, in combination, have contributed to the test score decline for more than the past fifteen years.

Efforts to end the decreases must address the curricular and school climate factors identified."

–Education Resources Center.gov

80 C3

U.S. ADHD Statistics

* 4.5 million children, 5-17 years of age have ever been diagnosed with ADHD as of 2006.

* 3%-7% of school-aged children suffer from ADHD. Some studies have estimated higher rates in community samples.

* 7.8% of school-aged children were reported to have an ADHD diagnosis by their parent in 2003. [see full article in reference section]

* Diagnosis of ADHD increased an average of 3% per year from 1997 to 2006. [see full article in reference section]

* Boys (9.5%) are more likely than girls (5.9%) to have been diagnosed with ADHD. [see full article]

* ADHD diagnosis is significantly higher among non-Hispanic, primarily English-speaking, and insured children. [see full article in reference section]

* Prevalence rates are significantly higher for children in families in which the most highly educated adult was a high school graduate (or had completed 12 years of education), compared with children in families in which the most highly educated adult had a higher or lower level of education. [see full article]

* ADHD diagnosis among males was reported significantly more often in families with incomes below the poverty threshold (<100%) than in families with incomes at or above the poverty threshold. Rates of reported diagnosis among females were not significantly different across the three levels of poverty. [see full article in reference section]

* Prevalence varies substantially by state, from a low of 5% in Colorado to a high of 11.1% in Alabama.

–Centers of Disease Control

ଞ୍ଚ ଓଷ

Student aptitude & learning decline

* American kids are good readers in comparison to many of their peers across the globe. Only three countries significantly outscored the U.S. at the elementary and high school levels (PIRLS, 2001; PISA 2000). The reading performance of our 4th graders was particularly strong. They scored significantly above the international average (PIRLS, 2001), while our 15-year-olds scored slightly above the average (PISA, 2000).

* Our math performance is mediocre. American 4th graders performed above the international average but were significantly outdone by young math students in 11 of the 25 nations participating in the assessment (TIMSS, 2003). Our 8th graders performed about the same (TIMSS, 2003). By high school, our students' performance falls below the international average. Only 11 of the 39 participating nations did significantly worse than the U.S. (PISA, 2003).

* U.S. science performance is a study of contrasts. On one hand, both American 4th and 8th-graders scored above the international average (TIMSS, 2003). Only three countries did significantly better than the U.S. with their elementary students, and American 4th-graders outperformed their counterparts in 16 other countries (TIMSS, 2003). But as in math, our high school students were significantly outscored in science by their peers in 18 of the 38 participating countries with a performance that was below the international average (PISA, 2003).

* The gap between affluent and poor students in the U.S. is near the international average. When comparing students' performance by parents' educational level, parents' occupation, and number of books in the home, Canada, Finland, and Iceland had smaller achievement

248

gaps than the U.S. while Germany had a larger gap (Hampden-Thompson and Johnston, 2006). The results are similar when looking at students by their immigration status and first language spoken.

* The American adult population (age 16 to 65) performed near the bottom on a six-nation assessment of literacy and numeracy. The U.S. performance exceeded only Italy's. Outscoring us were Norway, Bermuda, Canada, and Switzerland (ALL, 2003).

–The Center for Public Education

ಐ Oß

As we have seen, there is no clear answer for how well U.S. schools are doing compared to other countries. Contrary to some observers, U.S. students are not failing. But scores do show that other countries are doing better than the United States, even with similar groups of students.

Many analysts have noted that American fourth graders do relatively well on international tests, our eighth graders perform about average, and our older students fall beneath the international average. They suggest that this shows a relative decline in American school effectiveness (see for example, National Science Foundation, Science and Engineering Indicators 2000).

—The Center for Public Education

"During the past 20 years there has been a dramatic increase in obesity in the United States. In 2009, only Colorado and the District of Columbia had a prevalence of obesity less than 20%. Thirty-three states had a prevalence equal to or greater than 25%; nine of these states (Alabama, Arkansas, Kentucky, Louisiana, Mississippi, Missouri, Oklahoma, Tennessee, and West Virginia) had a prevalence of obesity equal to or greater than 30%."

—Centers for Disease Control

80 03

Reference

1.Student aptitude and learning

http://nces.ed.gov/programs/coe/press/highlights2.asp

2.The decline of literacy

http://onlinelibrary.wiley.com/doi/10.1111/j.1460-
2466.1980.tb01777.x/abstract

3.SAT scores show disparities by race, gender, family income. USA
Today

http://www.usatoday.com/news/education/2009-08-25-SAT-
scores_N.htm

4.Are we losing the race?

http://www.centerforpubliceducation.org/site/c.lvIXIiNOJwE/b.50
57297/k.3767/More_than_a_horse_race_A_guide_to_internation
al_tests_of_student_achievement.htm#losing_race_link

5.History-The Center for Public Education

http://www.centerforpubliceducation.org/site/apps/nlnet/conten
t3.aspx?c=lvIXIiNOJwE&b=5127791&ct=6857831&notoc=1

6.The decline of standardized test scores in the United States from
1965 to the Present.

http://www.eric.ed.gov/ERICWebPortal/search/detailmini.jsp?_nf
pb=true&_&ERICExtSearch_SearchValue_0=ED252565&ERICExtSe
arch_SearchType_0=no&accno=ED252565

7.Relationship between baseline glycemic control and cognitive
function in Individuals With Type 2 diabetes and other
cardiovascular risk factors
http://care.diabetesjournals.org/content/32/2/221.full

8.Diseases Transmitted Through Milk.; M.M. Kaplan, V.M.D.;
M.P.H.; M. Abdussalam, L.V.P.; Ph.D.; & G. Bijlenga
http://www.asmscience.org/content/book/10.1128/97815558184
63.chap29

9.Milk does a body good
http://www.westonaprice.org

10.   Disease escalation CDC + obesity prevalence maps
http://asmbs.org/wp/uploads/2014/05/Obesity-in-America.pdf
http://www.cdc.gov/obesity/data/prevalence-maps.html

11.Classifying obesity as a disease
http://health.usnews.com/health-
news/news/articles/2013/06/19/us-doctors-group-labels-obesity-
a-disease

12.YouTube video: High sugar diets and disease; Dr. Kimber
Stanhope; Department of Nutrition, U.C. Davis
https://www.youtube.com/watch?v=_AJka21yfyE

13. YouTube video: Fat, Fructose and FGF21- The science behind fad diets and obesity; Patricia Chui, MD; Department of Surgery, Grand Rounds, March 26, 2014
https://www.youtube.com/watch?v=YE4dlGrGPYk

14. Process food evolution
http://www.fda.gov/Food/IngredientsPackagingLabeling/GRAS/ucm094040.htm

15. Milk-borne infections. An analysis of their potential effect on the milk industry
http://www.ncbi.nlm.nih.gov/pmc/articles/PMC3882853/

16. Taste inflation revealed: why sugar, salt and fragrance make you stupid.
http://www.naturalnews.com/012556.html

17. U.S. Department of Education
http://nces.ed.gov/programs/coe/press/highlights2.asp

18. Thomas Fordham Institute – State of the States
http://www.edexcellence.net/detail/news.cfm?news_id=358

19. Sugar makes you stupider
http://www.raisin-hell.com/2009/02/sugar-makes-you-stupider.html

20. Attention-deficit / hyperactivity disorder (ADHD)
http://parentingteens.about.com/cs/addadhd/a/add_stats.htm

21. Baby food quality

http://www.naturalnews.com/012556.html

22. Diabetes in society

http://www.idf.org/diabetes-costs-hinder-economic-growth

23. Dietary guidelines for Americans, 2005

http://www.health.gov/dietaryguidelines/dga2005/document/pdf
/DGA2005.pdf

24. Nutrition labeling guide

http://www.fda.gov/Food/GuidanceComplianceRegulatoryInform
ation/GuidanceDocuments/FoodLabelingNutrition/FoodLabelingG
uide/ucm064894.htm

25. Sugar labeling

http://www.cspinet.org/new/fda_sugarlabeling.html

26. Center for Science in Public Interest - Nutrition action letter

http://www.fda.gov/OHRMS/DOCKETS/98fr/992630cp1.pdf

27. How much sugar do you really eat?

http://www.netdoctor.co.uk/dietandnutrition/toomuchsugar.htm

28. Global cancer facts and figures 2007

http://www.cancer.org/acs/groups/content/@nho/documents/do
cument/globalfactsandfigures2007rev2p.pdf

29. National vital statistics reports

http://www.cdc.gov/nchs/data/nvsr/nvsr57/nvsr57_14.pdf

30. Tobin, K. J. (2013), Fast-food consumption and educational test scores in the USA. Child: Care, Health and Development, 118–124. doi: 10.1111/j.1365-2214.2011.01349
http://onlinelibrary.wiley.com/doi/10.1111/j.1365-2214.2011.01349.x/abstract;jsessionid=09DA8FBF657F3AD496DB01A5F60AF1AD.f02t02

31. WHO - Causes of death worldwide
http://apps.who.int/gho/data/view.main.CODMDGDEVV

32. 2010 Updates American Heart Association
http://circ.ahajournals.org/cgi/reprint/CIRCULATIONAHA.109.192667

33. Dieting statistics. http://www.livestrong.com/article/438395-the-percentage-of-people-who-regain-weight-after-rapid-weight-loss-risks/

34. CDC Obesity Prevalence maps
http://www.cdc.gov/obesity/data/prevalence-maps.html

35. Advanced human nutrition
Http://health.jbpub.com/advancednutrition/Login.aspx?ref=/advancednutrition/default.aspx

36. Diet Industry worth 2014-2015
http://fortune.com/2015/05/22/lean-times-for-the-diet-industry/

37. Recycling the dead
https://student.societyforscience.org/article/recycling-dead

38. America's Greatest Health Threat: Obesity - Bloomberg, November 17, 2009

http://www.bloomberg.com/news/articles/2009-11-17/americas-greatest-health-threat-obesity

39. Almost 50% of people hospitalized for the flu are obese| Weise, USATODAY, January 13, 2014

http://www.usatoday.com/story/news/nation/2014/01/10/influenza-hospitalization-obese-h1n1/4409975/

40. Dementia Now Afflicting People in Their 40s as Mercury from Vaccines Causes Slow, Degenerative Brain Damage

http://www.realfarmacy.com/dementia-mercury-vaccines/

41. A.M.A. Recognizes Obesity as a Disease, Ney York Times, June 2013

http://www.nytimes.com/2013/06/19/business/ama-recognizes-obesity-as-a-disease.html?_r=0

42. Simple definition of Obesity. Harvard School of Public Health. T.H. Chan

https://www.hsph.harvard.edu/obesity-prevention-source/obesity-definition/

43. Page 23 additional statistics

Obesity: http://stateofobesity.org/healthcare-costs-obesity/

Food Industry: https://www.statista.com/topics/1660/food-retail/

Pharmaceutical Industry:

Https://www.statista.com/topics/1719/pharmaceutical-industry/

Resources

A final request:

Thank you for purchasing The Ingredient Diet.

Would you consider posting a favorable review on my
Amazon author page? In addition to providing feedback,
online reviews can help other customers learn about your
personal experience, and why this book offers a different
perspective on wellness and weight loss.

Please take a moment to rate the book and leave your
comments using the link below.

https://www.amazon.com/s/ref=nb_sb_noss?url=search-
alias%3Daps&field-
keywords=valerie+lunden&rh=i%3Aaps%2Ck%3Avalerie+lunden

Your support means a great deal to me.

With gratitude,

Valerie H. Lunden

INGREDIENT SHOPPING LIST - PORTABLE

Meat (all) Fresh, non hormone and pasture raised	Small and safe quantities of a daily probiotic (organic, coconut derived and Kombucha tea are good sources)
Fish (all) Consciously acquired/raised and non-hormone derived)	Non-ripened fruit. (organic) Buying smaller quantities helps manage this. 1-3 items each week
Vegetarian protein sources include legumes, pulses, organically produced soy products in limited quantities.	Vegetables (any; including starchy vegetables; undercooked, raw and organic)
Chocolate (dark/70% or more Cocoa, low sugar varieties)	Oils (always organic; not heat processed or over cooked; eaten for nutrition purposes)
Honey (organic, unprocessed and raw)	Coffee (organic brands and espresso, which has a lower acidity)
Milk Dairy (limited and consciously created) Produced by grass fed animals. No fillers or additives.	Tea (herbal and Kombucha) Multivitamins - Ethically produced, with no fillers. Research is recommended.
Eggs (unprocessed, raw and organic)	Organic coconut water.
Nuts (unprocessed, raw and organic)	
Seeds (unprocessed, raw and organic).	

ID Shopping List Reminders

Ingredient management is ALWAYS key.

Pick different foods each week to create variety, which limits food boredom.

Take advantage of the Nil day to enjoy more widespread ingredient recipes (this helps limit boredom).

Quantities are not restricted. Calories are limited to respectable daily intake needs.

Ingredients are always observed for quality and quantity. Solid foods are consumed when the eating window opens, which is after the body has completed digest its last cycle of food.

The following chart is divided into 2 sections, the first being more alkaline trending foods. To ensure a digestion-friendly blood chemistry, managing alkaline and acid ratios can also track the efficiency of enzymes, both in the mouth and stomach. In general, acid enzymes will work better on acid foods, and vice versa. Any combination of acids and alkaline foods slows digestion.

Alkaline forming foods = less acid performance during digestion.

Food Category	Food	Increased Alkalinity -->		
Dairy	Buttermilk	x		
Beverages	Tea (herbal, green)	x		
Beverages & Drinks	Water (most bottled varieties)	x		
Fats & Oils	Borage oil (not for cooking)	x		
Fats & Oils	**Coconut Oil (raw)**	x		
Fats & Oils	Evening Primrose oil (not for cooking)	x		
Fats & Oils	Flax seed oil (not for cooking)	x		
Fats & Oils	Marine lipids (not for cooking)	x		
Fats & Oils	Olive oil	x		
Fats & Oils	Sesame oil	x		
Fruits	Avocado (protein)		x	
Fruits	Banana (ripe)	x		
Fruits	**Banana (under ripe)**		x	
Fruits	Cherry, sour	x		
Fruits	Coconut, fresh	x		
Fruits	Figs (dried)	x		
Fruits	Figs (raw)	x		
Fruits	Fresh Lemon	x		
Fruits	Limes	x		

Fruits	Tomato	x		
Grains & Legumes	Buckwheat	x		
Grains & Legumes	Kamut	x		
Grains & Legumes	Lentils	x		
Grains & Legumes	Lima beans		x	
Grains & Legumes	Spelt	x		
Grains & Legumes	White (navy) beans		x	
Misc.	Baking soda		x	
Nuts	Almond (Organic)	x		
Nuts	Almond Butter (Organic) (Raw)	x		
Roots	Carrot	x		
Roots	Red Beet		x	
Roots	Potato	x		
Roots	Red radish		x	
Roots	Rutabaga	x		
Roots	Summer Black Radish			
Roots	Turnip	x		
Roots	Yams	x		
Seeds	Caraway seeds	x		
Seeds	Cumin seeds	x		
Seeds	Fennel seeds	x		
Seeds	Sesame seeds	x		
Vegetables	Alfalfa		x	
Vegetables	Artichokes	x		
Vegetables	Asparagus	x		
Vegetables	Egg plant	x		
Vegetables	Barley grass			
Vegetables	Basil	x		
Vegetables	Bell peppers/capsicums (all colors)	x		
Vegetables	Bok Choy	x		
Vegetables	Brussels sprouts	x		

Vegetables	Cabbage lettuce, fresh		x	
Vegetables	Cauliflower	x		
Vegetables	Cayenne pepper		x	
Vegetables	Celery		x	
Vegetables	Chives	x		
Vegetables	Cilantro		x	
Vegetables	Cucumber, fresh			
Vegetables	Dandelion			
Vegetables	Dog grass			
Vegetables	Endive, fresh		x	
Vegetables	French cut (green) beans		x	
Vegetables	Garlic		x	
Vegetables	Ginger		x	
Vegetables	Ginseng	x		
Vegetables	Green cabbage,	x		
Vegetables	Green cabbage,	x		
Vegetables	Horse radish	x		
Vegetables	Jicama			
Vegetables	Kale			
Vegetables	Kamut grass			
Vegetables	Lamb's lettuce	x		
Vegetables	Leeks	x		
Vegetables	Lettuce	x		
Vegetables	Mustard greens	x		
Vegetables	Onion	x		
Vegetables	Oregano		x	
Vegetables	Parsnips	x		
Vegetables	Peas, ripe	x		
Vegetables	Peppers	x		
Vegetables	Pumpkins (raw)	x		
Vegetables	Raw onions	x		
Vegetables	Red cabbage	x		
Vegetables	Rhubarb stalks	x		

Vegetables	Savoy Cabbage	x		
Vegetables	Sea Vegetables	x		
Vegetables	Seaweed	x		
Vegetables	Shave grass			
Vegetables	Sorrel		x	
Vegetables	Soy Sprouts			
Vegetables	Spinach	x		
Vegetables	Spinach		x	
Vegetables	Sprouted seeds (all kinds)			
Vegetables	Squash (all kinds)	x		
Vegetables	Straw grass			
Vegetables	Thyme	x		
Vegetables	Tomatoes (puree)	x		
Vegetables	Tomatoes (raw)	x		
Vegetables	Tomatoes (sundried)	x		
Vegetables	Watercress	x		
Vegetables	Wheat grass			
Vegetables	White cabbage	x		
Vegetables	Zucchini	x		
Organic varieties may have be slightly more alkaline.				

**Bold preferred.

Acid forming foods= less alkaline enzyme performance.

Food Category	Food	<-- Increased Acidity		
Breads	Corn Tortillas		x	
Breads	Rye bread			x
Breads	Sourdough bread		x	
Breads	White biscuit			x
Breads	White bread		x	
Breads	Whole-grain bread			x
Breads	Whole-meal bread			x
Condiments (most)	Ketchup, Mayonnaise, Miso, Mustard, Soy Sauce		x	
Dairy	Cheese (all varieties, from all milks)		x	
Dairy	Cream			x
Dairy	Eggs (whole or whites)		x	
Dairy	Homogenized and or Pasteurized Milk			x
Dairy	Yoghurt (all)			x
Beverages & Drinks	Beer	x		
Beverages & Drinks	Coffee	x		
Beverages & Drinks	Coffee substitute drinks			x
Beverages & Drinks	Fruit juice (natural)			x
Beverages & Drinks	Fruit juice (sweetened)	x		
Beverages & Drinks	Liquor	x		
Beverages & Drinks	Soda/Pop	x		
Beverages & Drinks	Tea (black)	x		
Beverages & Drinks	Water (sparkling)		x	
Beverages & Drinks	Water (spring)			x

Category	Item			
Beverages & Drinks	Wine		x	
Fats & Oils	Butter			x
Fats & Oils	Cod liver oil (not for cooking)			x
Fats & Oils	Corn oil			x
Fats & Oils	Margarine			x
Fats & Oils	Sunflower oil			x
Fruits	**Acai Berries**			x
Fruits	Apples			x
Fruits	Apricot			x
Fruits	Apricots			x
Fruits	Apricots (dried)			x
Fruits	**Banana (unripe)**			x
Fruits	Blackberries			x
Fruits	Blueberry			x
Fruits	Cantaloupe			x
Fruits	Cherry, sweet			x
Fruits	Clementine(s)			x
Fruits	**Cranberry**			x
Fruits	**Currant**			x
Fruits	Dates			x
Fruits	Dates (dried)			x
Fruits	Fig juice powder			x
Fruits	**Goji berries**			x
Fruits	**Gooseberry, ripe**			x
Fruits	**Grapefruit**			x
Fruits	Grapes (ripe)	x		
Fruits	Italian plum			x
Fruits	Mandarin orange		x	
Fruits	Mango			x
Fruits	Nectarine			x

Category	Item			
Fruits	Orange			x
Fruits	Papaya			x
Fruits	Peach			x
Fruits	Pear			x
Fruits	Pineapple		x	
Fruits	Pomegranate		x	
Fruits	Raspberry		x	
Fruits	Red currant			x
Fruits	Rose hips		x	
Fruits	Strawberries			x
Fruits	Strawberry			x
Fruits	Tangerine			x
Fruits	Watermelon			x
Grains & Legumes	Basmati rice			x
Grains & Legumes	Brown rice		x	
Grains & Legumes	Bulgur wheat			x
Grains & Legumes	Couscous			x
Grains & Legumes	Oats			x
Grains & Legumes	Rye bread			x
Grains & Legumes	Wheat		x	
Meat, Poultry & Fish	Beef	x		
Meat, Poultry & Fish	Buffalo		x	
Meat, Poultry & Fish	Chicken		x	
Meat, Poultry & Fish	Duck		x	
Meat, Poultry & Fish	Fresh water fish		x	
Meat, Poultry & Fish	Liver			x

Category	Food			
Meat, Poultry & Fish	Ocean fish		x	
Meat, Poultry & Fish	Organ meats			x
Meat, Poultry & Fish	Oysters			x
Meat, Poultry & Fish	Pork	x		
Meat, Poultry & Fish	Sardines (canned)	x		
Meat, Poultry & Fish	Shrimp			x
Meat, Poultry & Fish	Tuna (canned)	x		
Meat, Poultry & Fish	Veal	x		
Meat, Poultry & Fish	Wild salmon,		x	
Misc	Apple Cider Vinegar			x
Misc	Canned foods		x	
Misc	Cereals		x	
Misc	Hummus			x
Misc	POPCORN			x
Misc	Rice milk			x
Misc	Soy Protein Powder			x
Misc	Whey protein powder			x
Nuts	Brazil nuts			x
Nuts	Cashews			x
Nuts	Filberts			x
Nuts	Hazelnut			x
Nuts	Macadamia nuts (raw)			x
Nuts	Peanut butter (raw, organic)		x	
Nuts	Peanuts		x	
Nuts	Pistachios		x	
Nuts	Walnuts			x
Roots	Sweet Potato			x
Seeds	Barley			x
Seeds	Flax seeds			x
Seeds	Pumpkin seeds			x

Seeds	Sunflower seeds			x
Seeds	Wheat Kernel	x		
Sweets & Sweeteners	Agave nectar			x
Sweets & Sweeteners	Alcohol sugars (including Xylitol)		x	
Sweets & Sweeteners	Artificial sweeteners	x		
Sweets & Sweeteners	Barley malt syrup			x
Sweets & Sweeteners	Beet sugar		x	
Sweets & Sweeteners	Brown rice syrup			x
Sweets & Sweeteners	Chocolates		x	
Sweets & Sweeteners	Dried sugarcane juice			x
Sweets & Sweeteners	Fructose			x
Sweets & Sweeteners	Halva [ground sesame seed sweet]		x	
Sweets & Sweeteners	Honey			x
Sweets & Sweeteners	Maple Syrup			x
Sweets & Sweeteners	Milk sugar			x
Sweets & Sweeteners	Molasses		x	
Sweets & Sweeteners	Sugar (white)		x	
Sweets & Sweeteners	Sugarcane		x	
Sweets & Sweeteners	Turbinado sugar			x
Sweets & Sweeteners	Xylitol		x	
Vegetables	Blue-Green Algae			x
Vegetables	Canned vegetables		x	
Vegetables	Cooked vegetables (all kinds)			x

Vegetables	Frozen vegetables		x	
Vegetables	Mushrooms		x	
Vegetables	Pickled vegetables	x		
Vegetables	Yeast			x
Organic varieties may be slightly more alkaline.				

**Bold options preferred

ID Schedule Tracker - Make Copies						
Date	**120 days or 6 week - Cycle #**					**Health Goals**
Weight	**Record after two 6-week cycles. The customizable schedule below is offered as a guide.** **List your schedule below.**					
Sample Schedule						
Sun	Mon	Tues	Wed	Thurs	Fri	Sat
Eating window ends after 3:00 PM	Eating window begins after 2:00 PM	Eating window begins after 2:00 PM	Eating window begins after 2:00 PM	Eating window ends after 3:00 PM	Eating window begins after 2:00 PM	Eating window begins after 2:00 PM
Potential free day	Eating window ends between 8-9 PM	Eating window ends between 8-9 PM	Eating window ends between 8-9 PM	Potential free day	Eating window ends between 8-9 PM	Eating window ends between 8-9 PM
My schedule						
Sun	Mon	Tues	Wed	Thurs	Fri	Sat

ID Schedule Tracker- Make Copies							
Date	120 days or 6 week - Cycle #						Health Goals
Weight	Record after two 6-week cycles. The customizable schedule below is offered as a guide. List your schedule below.						
Sample Schedule							
Sun	Mon	Tues	Wed	Thurs	Fri	Sat	
Eating window ends after 3:00 PM	Eating window begins after 2:00 PM	Eating window begins after 2:00 PM	Eating window begins after 2:00 PM	Eating window ends after 3:00 PM	Eating window begins after 2:00 PM	Eating window begins after 2:00 PM	
Potential free day	Eating window ends between 8-9 PM	Eating window ends between 8-9 PM	Eating window ends between 8-9 PM	Potential free day	Eating window ends between 8-9 PM	Eating window ends between 8-9 PM	
My schedule							
Sun	Mon	Tues	Wed	Thurs	Fri	Sat	

ID Weight Loss and Wellness Tracker (recorded weekly)

Date	Weight	Fat (fat monitoring scale)	ID Week #

Overall Wellness Tracker (recorded every 6 months)

Date	Cholesterol	Glucose	pH

ID Weight Loss and Wellness Tracker (recorded weekly)

Date	Weight	Fat (fat monitoring scale)	ID Week #

Overall Wellness Tracker (recorded every 6 months)

Date	Cholesterol	Glucose	pH

ID Weight Loss and Wellness Tracker (recorded weekly)

Date	Weight	Fat (fat monitoring scale)	ID Week #

Overall Wellness Tracker (recorded every 6 months)

Date	Cholesterol	Glucose	pH

ID Weight Loss and Wellness Tracker (recorded weekly)

Date	Weight	Fat (fat monitoring scale)	ID Week #

Overall Wellness Tracker (recorded every 6 months)

Date	Cholesterol	Glucose	pH

ID Weight Loss and Wellness Tracker (recorded weekly)			
Date	Weight	Fat (fat monitoring scale)	ID Week #

Overall Wellness Tracker (recorded every 6 months)			
Date	Cholesterol	Glucose	pH

ID Weight Loss and Wellness Tracker (recorded weekly)

Date	Weight	Fat (fat monitoring scale)	ID Week #

Overall Wellness Tracker (recorded every 6 months)

Date	Cholesterol	Glucose	pH

Obesity Trends* Among U.S. Adults
BRFSS, 1985

(*BMI ≥30, or ~ 30 lbs. overweight for 5' 4" person)

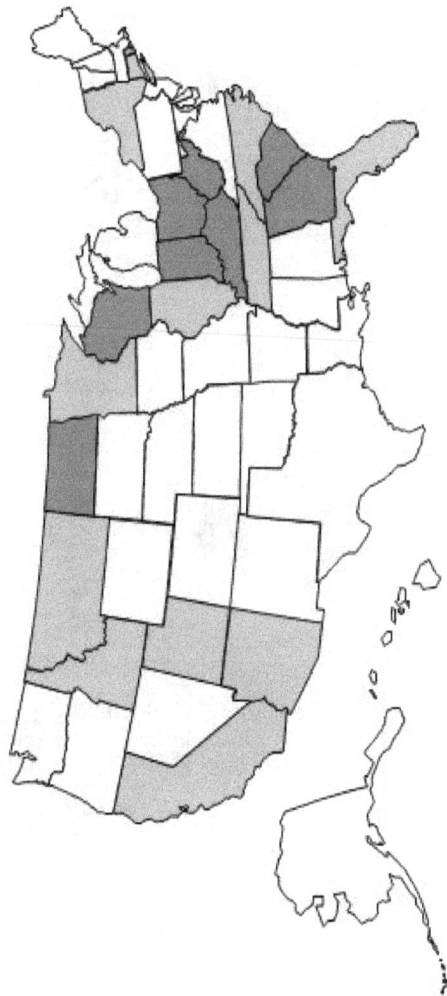

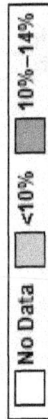

No Data   <10%   10%–14%

Source: Behavioral Risk Factor Surveillance System, CDC.

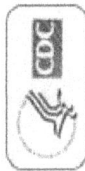

Obesity Trends* Among U.S. Adults
BRFSS, 1990

(*BMI ≧30, or ~ 30 lbs. overweight for 5' 4" person)

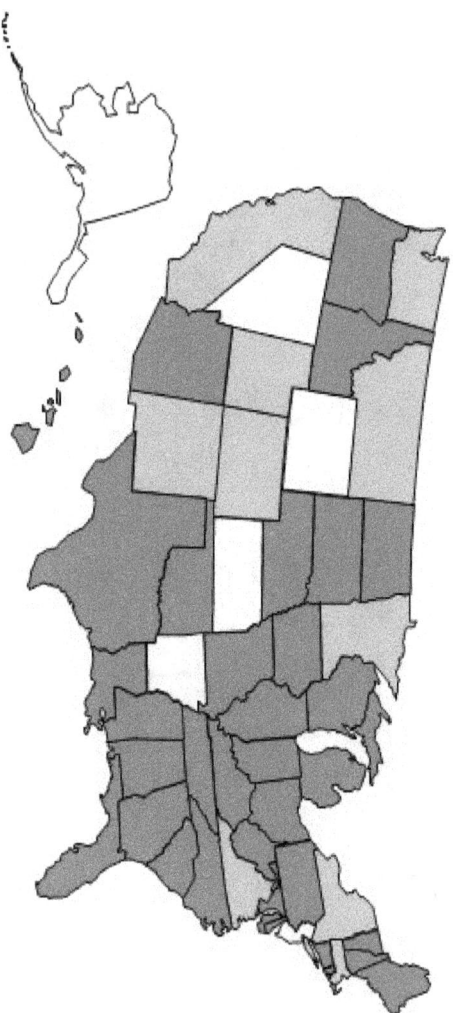

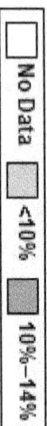

No Data

<10%

10%–14%

Source: Behavioral Risk Factor Surveillance System, CDC.

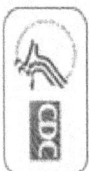

Obesity Trends* Among U.S. Adults
BRFSS, 2010

(*BMI ≥30, or ~ 30 lbs. overweight for 5′ 4″ person)

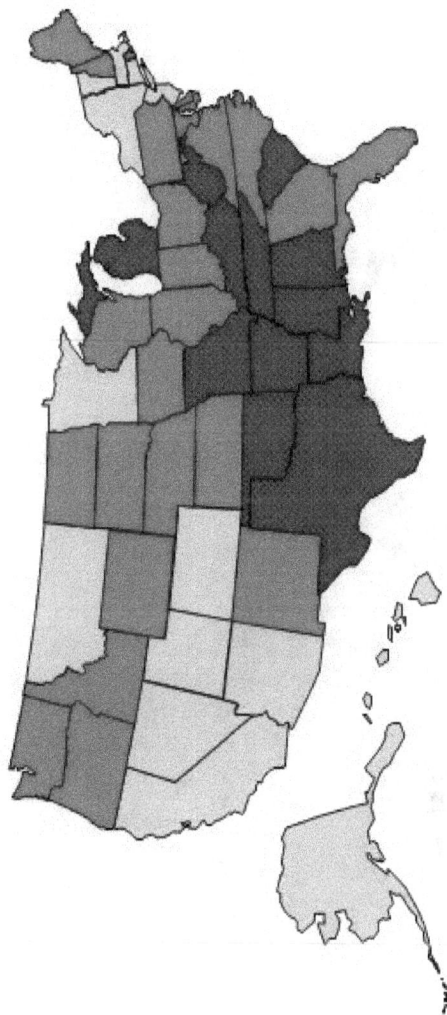

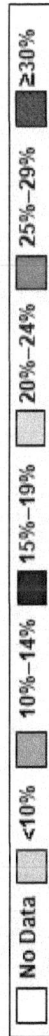

No Data   <10%   10%–14%   15%–19%   20%–24%   25%–29%   ≥30%

Source: Behavioral Risk Factor Surveillance System, CDC.

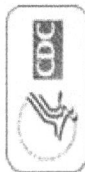

Prevalence[1] of Self-Reported Obesity Among U.S. Adults by State and Territory, BRFSS, 2014

[1] Prevalence estimates reflect BRFSS methodological changes started in 2011. These estimates should not be compared to prevalence estimates before 2011.

*Sample size <50 or the relative standard error (dividing the standard error by the prevalence) ≥ 30%.

Legend:
- <20%
- 20%–<25%
- 25%–<30%
- 30%–<35%
- ≥35%
- No data available*

Health & Weight Loss Companion

Why we repeat old food behaviors, disrupt weight loss and avoid better health.

VALERIE H. LUNDEN, M.A.

Health & Weight Loss Companion
Everyday Journal

INCLUDES EXTRA BONUS SECTION

- Manage & Improve Health Focus
- Build Continuous Motivation
- Identify Food Beliefs & Behaviors
- Realize Positive Wellness Opportunities

VALERIE H. LUNDEN, M.A.

HIS INCOMPARABLE DUCHESS

V. H. Lunden

Customer Service Handbook

VALERIE H. LUNDEN, M.A.

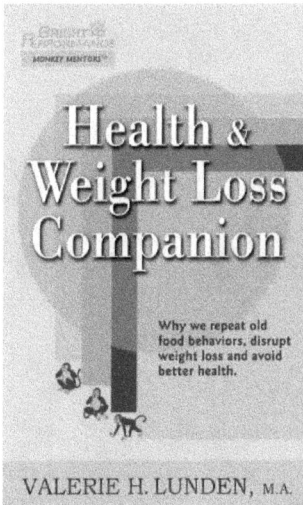

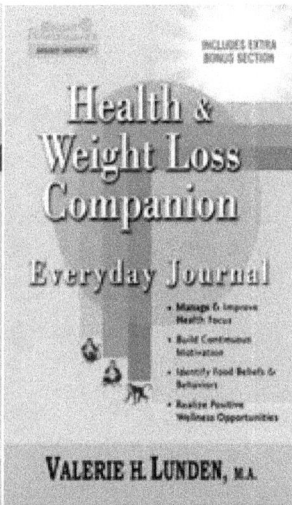

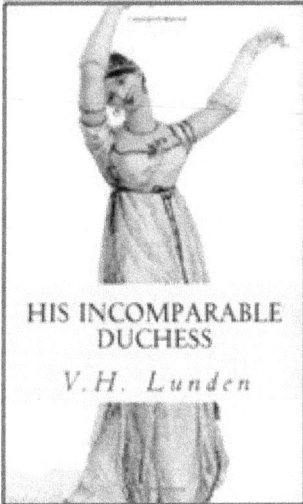

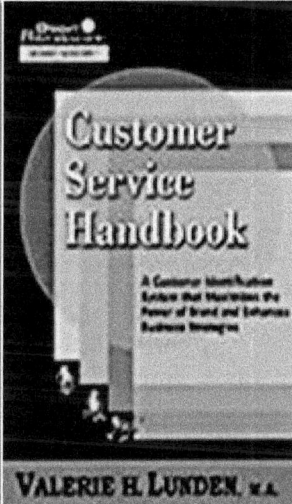

About the Author

Valerie H. Lunden is an idea's person. She writes and creates based on her compelling interest in all questions unanswered. Whether her invention is a health premise or a tasty (and healthy) surprise, her inspired imagination continues to explore. Valerie is the recipient of a master's degree in creative writing, and an undergraduate degree in business.

More of Valerie's books are available at
www.valsden.com

www.ingramcontent.com/pod-product-compliance
Lightning Source LLC
Chambersburg PA
CBHW062202270326
41930CB00009B/1617